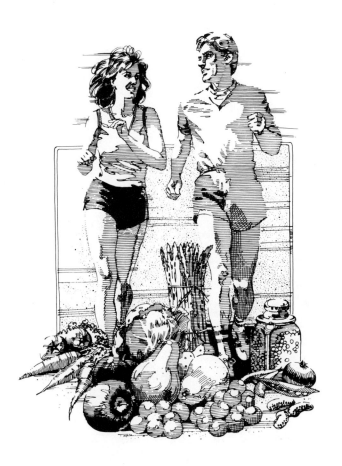

GETTING IN SHAPE

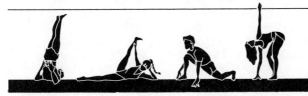

Cindy Pemberton
M.P.H., R.D.

*All recipes have been tested and approved
by Chris Weahunt, R.D.*

Creative Arts Book Company

Berkeley, California • 1983

Creative Arts Book Company
833 Bancroft Street
Berkeley, CA 94710

ISBN 0-916870-68-5

Library of Congress Catalogue
Card Number 83-072832

The text for *Getting In Shape* was set in 10/11 Garamond by Green Valley Graphics, Placerville, California.

To my love,
Roy

FOREWORD

Evidence is everywhere of the growing interest in and commitment to physical fitness and good nutrition. As individuals and as a nation, we have realized the physical and psychological benefits that a sensible nutrition and fitness program can provide. Research shows that a sound diet and daily exercise are the means to excellent health. Exercise and good nutrition lower the incidence of many diseases, including hypertension, heart disease, and many types of cancer. But equally important, a good fitness program makes you *feel* better, and improves your outlook on life.

Getting in shape is a matter of *both* exercise and diet. Cindy Pemberton's book provides all you need to quickly and easily begin your own personal fitness program. it is filled with sensible, simply-presented information on the basic aspects of nutrition, exercise, and weight loss. Anyone who makes use of this book will find it easy to achieve and maintain good health.

Lorelei Groll Ed.D., R.D.
Assistant Professor of Public Health Nutrition
School of Public Health,
University of California, Berkeley

INTRODUCTION

This book is for anyone who is interested in becoming fit—and staying that way. *Getting in Shape* is appropriate for females and males of all ages and all levels of fitness.

Most importantly, this book for people who are interested in DOING something about their life-style. *Getting in Shape* is an action-oriented book for DOERS instead of WANTERS. So if you're a doer, this book is the one for you.

Embarking on a fitness program and a new life-style means that diet and exercise must become top priorities. Excuses for not eating right or not exercising must wane. People can always find a reason to not do some physical activity or eat wholesome foods. THE DECISION must be made that time and effort will be set aside regularly for GETTING IN SHAPE and REMAINING IN SHAPE.

I hope you find this book informative and motivating. Here's to your new fitness program and your new life-style. I know you'll find them both fun and rewarding. Being in shape feels sooooo good!

—*Cindy Pemberton*

CONTENTS

1 FITNESS

People are becoming increasingly interested in the topic of FITNESS and becoming FIT. What does it mean to be "fit" or "in shape"? Often people think it means losing weight. If you're thin you've got to be fit—right? WRONG!

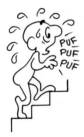

Thin people can be very out of shape! They can huff and puff going up stairs or taking a bicycle trip. They can run out of gas doing relatively simple activities.

There are also many people with loads of muscles who are out of shape. They can lift heavy objects with no problem. However, if you ask them to join you for a brisk walk or a swim in the lake, they tire out real fast.

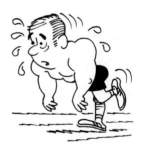

BODY WEIGHT

People who are fit do not tire easily during physical activity. The reasons for this are that they have:

(1) a low percentage of body fat;

(2) a high percentage of lean body tissue (muscle tissue); and

(3) a "conditioned" cardiovascular system (see page 45).

What you weigh on the scale is actually lean body tissue plus fat cells. That is:

Total body weight = lean body weight + fat weight

Lean body weight is composed of what's left over after body fat is removed: muscle, skin, bones, organs. Muscle tissue is very dense, body fat is not. Someone who floats with ease in a swimming pool has a lot of body fat. The person who sinks to the bottom has a low percentage of body fat.

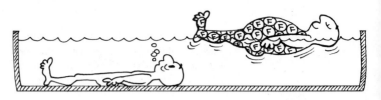

While body fat must be carried around with you, it does not contribute to your movement. Body fat is not metabolically active tissue. Your fat cells are free-loaders. You have to lug them around with you, but they don't help out. This extra work tires you quickly!

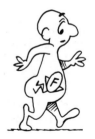

Lean body tissues—muscles—are the powerhouses of your body. They are very metabolically active, consuming oxygen and fuel, yielding strength and endurance.

Muscle tissue makes your body look lean and firm. Fat tissue is flabby and often jiggles when you run!

Muscles help you glide up a flight of stairs; body fat weighs you down as you go up each step.

There are benefits to having a BODY with a low percentage of body fat and a well-conditioned cardiovascular system. You can engage in the activities you want to with minimal effort. If you want to ride a bike, you get on it and go! If you need to run to catch a bus, you "kick into high gear" and take off. Being in shape, being fit, allows you to engage in most forms of physical activity without a second thought. It frees you to be as active as you want to be, thereby helping you to enjoy life. Fit people often find themselves:

- skiing
- running
- rowing
- cycling
- playing racquetball
- playing volleyball
- playing tennis
- flying a kite
- throwing a frisbee
- swimming
- taking walks
- taking hikes
- dancing
- moving

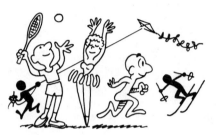

LOSING WEIGHT

If you are overfat (overweight), then a healthy change would be to lose some fat tissue and gain some lean body tissue.

Females should have approximately 14 to 25 percent body fat. The ideal body fat for women is about 18 percent. Males should have approximately 10 to 19 percent body fat. The ideal body fat for males is about 12 percent. (You can obtain your percentage of body fat by being weighed under water or using skinfold calipers. Most hospitals and sport medicine clinics have the proper tanks for underwater weighing.)

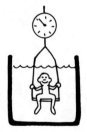

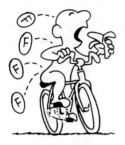

How do you lose body fat and maintain your lean body tissue? By eating a proper diet *and* exercising. When people lose weight by dieting only, they lose lean body tissue as well as fat tissue. However, when people both exercise and reduce their caloric intake, they lose mostly fat tissue.

In the following chapters you will learn how to eat properly, and how to get started in an exercise program that is right for you. Remember, getting in shape means *DOING*—it's action. Getting fit and staying fit means changing old habits and adopting new ones. It is a slow, gradual process—but a sure process. You'll get the hang of it, and once you do, LOOK OUT! Eating right and exercising regularly can be addictive. They lead to a very rewarding life-style, one that makes you feel good about yourself.

GETTING IN SHAPE takes

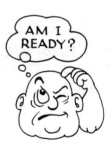

- Deciding that YOU want to be fit.
- Eating FREE foods (see the next chapter).
- Eating LESS.
- Exercising MORE.
- Keeping BUSY.

2 CALORIES IN FOOD

Losing body fat requires a COMMITMENT to a certain way of eating—a healthy way of eating. This means eating mainly foods that are LOW in FAT and SUGAR.

Foods that are high in fat or sugar are generally high in calories. (Calories measure how much energy there is in food.) If you eat lots of calories, you GAIN weight. If you eat only a few calories, you LOSE weight.

Some examples of high-fat foods include pizza, butter, oil, mayonnaise and salad dressing. Foods high in both fat and sugar include ice cream, cookies, cakes, and doughnuts. This does not mean that you have to ELIMI-NATE these foods entirely from your diet—it means that you eat these foods only occasionally.

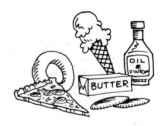

THE FOUR CALORIC GROUPS

Based on CALORIES there are four food groups:

■ **Free Foods:** They are so low in calores that you can fill up on them!

■ **Light Foods:** They have about half as many calories per bite as

■ **Heavy Foods,** which are generally high in fat and/or sugar.

- **Junk Foods:** They are high in calories, and provide little if any nutrients. You want to DE-EMPHASIZE these foods in your diet.

The only foods that you can eat in large amounts and still lose weight are FREE FOODS. The amount of food you eat from the other groups affects your weight. Therefore, eat SMALL or AVERAGE portions of food. For example:

- One banana, not two
- One scoop of rice, not two
- One sandwich, not two

(For average portion sizes, see the Exchange List on page 11.)

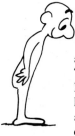 CAREFULLY look at the following food chart and see which FREE and LIGHT foods you enjoy. Then go to the grocery store and stock up on them! It is PARAMOUNT that you have these foods on hand, so that when you get hungry they are readily available. This may seem like a small, simple concept, but it is a KEY CONCEPT for weight reduction. You must not run out of the foods on your "food plan." Remember, FREE foods will not affect your weight, and LIGHT foods can when eaten in large quantities. HEAVY FOODS and JUNK FOODS can put on the pounds fast! Therefore, eating small or average portions of LIGHT foods is MUCH BETTER than eating HEAVY and JUNK FOODS.

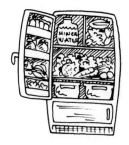

FOODS IN THE
FOUR CALORIC GROUPS

Asterisks indicate foods high in salt or sodium.

Free Foods

Alfalfa sprouts
Artichokes
Asparagus
Broccoli
Brussels sprouts
Mushrooms
Herbs and spices
Cabbage
Carrots, raw
Cauliflower
Celery
Cucumber
Eggplant
Green beans
Green onions
Green pepper
Greens
Lettuce

Jicama
Onions
Radishes
Spinach
Sunchokes
Tomatoes
Zucchini
Carrots
Low-calorie dressing*
Mineral water
Vegetable juice*
Lemon
Lime
Vinegar
Coffee
Tea
Diet soda*

Light Foods

Nonfat milk
Low-fat milk
Buttermilk
Plain yogurt
Cottage cheese*
Fish
Shellfish
Chicken (no skin)
Turkey
Beans (no fat/sugar)

Strawberries
Pineapple
Oranges
Corn
Winter squash
Yams
Mixed vegetables
Potatoes
Peas
Whole wheat bread

Tofu
Tempeh
Apples
Bananas
Peaches
Grapes
Grapefruit

Plain popcorn
Puffed wheat
Corn tortillas
Rye crackers
Oatmeal
Barley
Brown rice

Heavy Foods

Whole milk
Flavored Yogurt
Cheese*
Beef, Lamb, Pork
Ham,* Bacon*
Luncheon meats*
Sausage,* Salami*
Fish sticks*
Hot dogs*
Hamburgers
TV dinners*
Tacos*
Burritos*
Pizza*
Creamed Soups*
Avocado

Peanut butter
Raisins
Canned fruit
Biscuits
Sweet muffins
Waffles
Pancakes
French toast
Coffee cake
Sweetened cereals
Bulgur
Fried rice
Snack crackers*
Casseroles
Cornbread

Junk Foods

Cake
Candy
Cookies
Pie
Doughnuts
Sweet rolls
Shakes
Sodas
Kool Aid
Potato chips*
Corn chips*

French fries*
Onion rings*
Cream cheese
Ice cream
Salad dressing
Sherbert
Pudding
Butter, Margarine
Oil
Mayonnaise

3 THE EXCHANGE SYSTEM

Instead of using the General Guidelines on free, light, heavy, and junk foods, some people prefer to know how many calories they are eating each day. Women can generally eat **1200 calories** each day and lose weight. Men can eat **1500 calories** each day and

Daily Intake	
Women	1200 Calories
Men	1500 Calories

lose weight. There are those who have to eat only *700 to 1000 calories* daily and lose weight at a safe rate. If you are not losing 1 to 2 pounds each week on a 1200-calorie food plan, then lower your caloric intake by a couple of hundred calories (2 servings of bread or 4 servings of fat). An EASY way to keep track of calories is by using the *EXCHANGE SYSTEM*.

Food can be broken down into six categories: starch, vegetables, fruit, protein, milk, and fat. Most foods within the same food group **are** approximately the same in calories:

the calories in one apple =
the calories in one pear =
the calories in one small banana =
the calories in one peach.

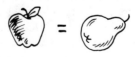

The same is true for protein-rich foods:

the calories in one ounce of fish =
the calories in one ounce of poultry =
the calories in one ounce of shellfish.

The system for substituting foods within the same food group, leaving the calorie and nutrient content about the same, has been labeled the EXCHANGE SYSTEM: an apple can be exchanged for a pear, 2 ounces of chicken can be exchanged for 2 ounces of shrimp, and so on.

The STARCH GROUP contains breads, cereals, and starchy vegetables. A potato can be exchanged for a slice of bread or a half cup of hot cereal. By substituting one for the other, the calorie count will not be altered.

The FAT GROUP contains nuts, oils, avocados, and bacon. (Bacon is so fatty it is not considered a protein, but rather a fat!) One slice of bacon is equivalent in calories and fat to one teaspoon of butter or eight almonds.

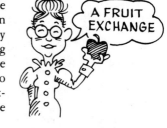

In the world of nutrition, foods are often called exchanges. A dietitian who has been on the job too long may explain her menu in the following manner: "I ate one fruit exchange (an apple), two bread exchanges (two slices of toast), and three fat exchanges (two pats of butter and one strip bacon)—great meal!"

It is important to point out that the stated caloric content of any food is **approximation**. That is, the number of calories in one apple will vary some from the number found in another.

An apple will also be digested differently by different people. Some people absorb more food from their digestive tract, and therefore more calories, than others. For example, if two people are eating an 80-calorie apple, one person may absorb only 75 calories from that apple, and another may absorb only 60 calories.

The degree of refinement of the food determines how much you will absorb. The more refined the food, the more you absorb. Thus, **whole-grain** products are good to eat because they leave some residue in your digestive tract. However, **white-enriched** products leave hardly any. It is better to emphasize unrefined foods in your diet, which are high in fiber (bulk). YOUR BODY IS NOT SUPPOSED TO ABSORB ALL THE FOOD YOU EAT.

Whole foods are better for you from more than just the standpoint of calories. The fiber found in unprocessed foods seems to help reduce the risk of developing colon cancer, diverticulosis, diabetes, and heart disease. (For a list of unrefined, wholesome foods, see page 26.)

The chart that follows gives the calorie content of foods in the different food groups. Remember, people need a WIDE VARIETY of foods in their diet. So, select different foods from each group—and enjoy!

THE STARCH GROUP— BREAD, GRAIN, AND STARCHY VEGETABLES

EACH BREAD, GRAIN, AND STARCHY VEGETABLE = IS ONE 70-CALORIE SERVING.

Bagel	1/2
Beans, dried, cooked	1/3 cup
Bread, whole wheat, rye, sourdough	1 slice
Cereal, hot, cracked wheat, oatmeal, Wheatena	1/2 cup
Cereal, cold, unsweetened flakes puffed	1 cup 1-1/2 cups

Corn on the cob	1 small (5" long)
Grapenuts cereal	1/4 cup
Kasha (buckwheat)	1/2 cup
Lentils, cooked	1/3 cup
Lima beans	1/3 cup
Muffin	1/2
Parsnips	1 small, 2/3 cup
Pasta	1/2 cup
Peas, black-eyed, split, cooked	1/3 cup
Peas, green, fresh or frozen	2/3 cup
Pita, whole wheat	1/2 of a 6" pocket
Popcorn, air blown	3 cups cooked
Potatoes, white, mashed	1/2 cup
Potatoes, white, baked or broiled	1 small
Pumpkin, cooked	1/2 cup
Rice, brown, cooked	1/3 cup
Rice cakes	2
Rolls	1/2
Rye-Crisp, unseasoned	3 crackers
Shredded wheat cereal	1 large biscuit
Tortilla, corn	1"-6" in diameter
Winter squash, baked	1/2 cup
Yams, baked	1/4 cup

VEGETABLE GROUP

EACH VEGETABLE EXCHANGE = ONE 25-CALORIE SERVING.

Alfalfa sprouts	1 cup
Artichokes	1
Asparagus	8 spears
Bamboo shoots	1/2 cup
Beets	1/2 cup
Green beans	3/4 cup
Green and red bell pepper	1
Beet greens, cooked	1 cup
Broccoli	1/2 cup or 1/2 stalk

Brussels sprouts	1/2 cup
Cabbage	1 cup
Carrot	1 medium
Cauliflower	1 cup
Celery	1 cup, chopped
Swiss chard, cooked	1 cup
Cucumber	1 medium
Eggplant	3/4 cup
Lettuce	2-1/2 cups
Mushrooms	1 cup
Onions	1/2 cup
Parsnips	1/2 cup
Pea pods	1/2 cup
Rutabaga	1/2 cup
Spinach, raw	2 cups
Summer Squash	1 cup
Tomato	1
Tomato paste	2 Tbsp.
Tomato juice	1/2 cup
Tomatoe puree	1/4 cup
Turnips, raw	1 cup
Turnip greens, cooked	1 cup
Water chestnuts	5

FRUIT GROUP

EACH FRUIT EXCHANGE = ONE 40-CALORIE SERVING.

Apple	1 small
Apricots	2 medium
Banana	1/2 large
Berries (boysenberries, blackberries, rasberries, blueberries)	3/4 cup
Cantaloupe	1/4
Cherries	10 large (1/2 cup)
Fig, fresh	1 large
Grapefruit	1/2 small

Grapes	12 large (1/2 cup)
Honeydew melon	1/4
Mango	1/2 small
Nectarine	1 medium
Orange	1 small
Papaya	1/3 medium (3/4 cup)
Peach	1 medium
Pear	1 small
Persimmon	1/2 medium
Pineapple	1/2 cup
Plums	2 medium
Pomegranate	1 small
Strawberries	3/4 cup
Tangarine	1 large
Watermelon	3/4 cup

MILK GROUP

EACH MILK EXCHANGE = ONE 90-CALORIE SERVING.

Nonfat milk	1 cup
Nonfat dry milk powder	1/3 cup
Low-fat milk	2/3 cup (or 1 cup and omit 1 fat from your diet)
Whole milk	1/2 cup (or 1 cup and omit 2 fats from your diet)
Buttermilk	1 cup
Nonfat yogurt, plain	2/3 cup
Low-fat yogurt	1/2 cup (or 2/3 cup and omit 1 fat from your diet)

PROTEIN GROUP

EACH LEAN PROTEIN EXCHANGE = ONE 55-CALORIE SERVING.

Fish	1 oz.
Tuna packed in water	1/4 cup
Shellfish	1/4 cup
Scallops	5
Poultry (no skin)	1 oz.
Rabbit	1 oz.
Veal loin, round or shoulder	1 oz.
Beef round, trimmed	1 oz.
Dried beans or peas, cooked	1/3 cup
Cottage cheese	1/4 cup

EACH MEDIUM-FAT PROTEIN EXCHANGE = ONE 78-CALORIE SERVING.

Completely trimmed:	
Beef or veal	1 oz.
Lamb	1 oz.
Fresh ham	
Organ meats	1 oz.
Egg	1

EACH HIGH-FAT PROTEIN EXCHANGE = ONE 100-CALORIE SERVING.

Partially trimmed:	
Beef	1 oz.
Veal	1 oz.
Lamb	1 oz.
Pork	1 oz.
Luncheon meats	1 slice
Hot dogs	1
Hard cheese	1 oz.

Completely trimmed:
    Pork loin   1 oz.
    Ground beef   1 oz.
    Spareribs   1 oz.
    Veal cutlet   1 oz.

FAT GROUP

EACH FAT EXCHANGE = ONE 45-CALORIE SERVING.

Butter, Margarine	1 tsp.
Mayonnaise	1 tsp.
Oil	1 tsp.
Salad dressing, all types	1-1/2 tsp.
Avocado	1/8
Peanuts	10
Peanut Butter	2 tsp.
Walnuts	4-5 halves
Almonds	8
Sunflower seeds	1 Tbsp.
Sour cream	1-1/2 tsp.
Half and half	2 Tbsp.
Cream cheese	1 Tbsp.
Olives	5
Bacon	1 slice

MENU PLAN

The following chart gives you a possible menu plan, based on the Exchange System, for your daily diet. If you are on a 1200-calorie food plan, you can have two exchanges from the milk group. For example, you might want 1 cup of nonfat milk on your cereal for breakfast and 2/3 cup nonfat yogurt with your fresh fruit salad at lunch. Since your protein allotment is 6 exchanges, you may want an egg (1 exchange) with breakfast, 1/2 cup tuna (2 oz. = 2 exchanges) at lunch, and 3/4 cup shrimp (3 oz. = 3 exchanges) at dinner time. Or you may want to save all 6 oz. for a special crab feed.

Number of Exchanges

Foods	1000 Calories	1200 Calories	1500 Calories
Starches	3	5	6
Vegetables	2	2	3
Fruit	3	3	5
Milk	2	2	2
Protein	6	6	6
Fats	2	2	4

You can devise your own food plan as you eat throughout the day. Keep track of the various exchanges and then calculate the calorie count.

Here is an example, based on lunch of a peanut butter sandwich, an apple, and a cup of coffee.

■ One sandwich has 2 slices of bread, which
  = 2 bread exchanges,
  or 140 calories (70 calories x 2).

■ The 4 teaspoons of peanut butter
  = 2 fat exchanges,
  or 90 calories (45 calories x 2).

■ Add an apple, which
  = 1 fruit exchange,
  or 40 calories.

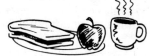

■ Coffee has no calories.

■ This adds up to: 2 bread exchanges
  2 fat exhanges
  1 fruit exchange.
  Total: 270 calories

If this lunch was eaten by a female on a 1200-calorie food plan, she could not consume ANY MORE FAT for the rest of the day (see the MENU PLAN on page 17). She has used up her quota of fat. On the bright side, though, her dinner might consist of a chicken breast baked in wine and garlic, a tossed green salad with low-fat Italian dressing, and a baked potato covered with mushrooms, green onions, tomatoes, and bell peppers (cooked *au naturel*). Not bad for a "fatless" dinner.

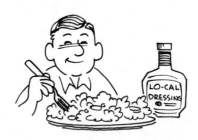

See the Calorie Chart (page 77) for some common foods not on the Exchange List. Be sure you don't go over your daily calorie quota that enables you to lose 1 to 2 pounds per week. Whatever that figure is, then STOP EATING when you've consumed your allotment! If you must eat, then eat ONLY FREE FOODS! (See page 7.)

Be sure to avoid some common bad habits:

- Don't eat snack foods instead of healthy foods—fruit, vegetables, milk, etc.—because your body needs the vitamins, minerals, and fiber found in wholesome foods.

- Don't save your calories for the last meal of the day. Your body can use only so many calories at one time. Since excess calories get shunted into fat, it is better to spread your calories out over the entire day:
  300 calories for breakfast
  400 calories for lunch
  400 calories for dinner
  100 calories for late-night snack.

4 NUTRITION

Besides CALORIES, food contains NUTRIENTS—chemical substances needed by our bodies to function properly. The major nutrient categories are protein, carbohydrates, fat, vitamins, minerals, water, and fiber (bulk). No single food or food group can supply all the essential nutrients needed to maintain good health. Therefore, it is important to eat a WIDE VARIETY of foods.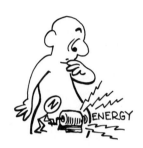

On the basis of their similar nutrient content, foods may be classified into groups. Each group makes special contributions to a nutritionally sound diet.

Listed below are six NUTRIENT food groups, assembled a little differently than the EXCHANGE groups in the previous chapter. For optimal nutrition, eat at least the number of servings listed for each nutrition group. This will equal about 1200 calories a day. You can use this as a DAILY guide for planning your meals.

PROTEIN is necessary for tissue maintenance and growth. Enzymes, hormones, and antibodies are mostly protein. Protein foods are a good source of B vitamins, iron, and zinc.

Serving size
Beans, 1/2 cup as side dish; 1 cup as main dish
Nuts, 1/4-1/2 cup
Peanut butter, 2-4 Tbsp.
Eggs, 1-2
Chicken, Fish, Meat, 2 oz.

19

Minimum Daily Serving: 2

- Light and heavy foods
- 45-100 calories per exchange
- Protein and fat exchange group

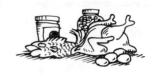

MILK AND MILK PRODUCTS are the best food sources of calcium. Calcium is necessary for proper bone mineralization and nerve transmission. Milk also contains protein, B vitamins, and vitamins A and D.

Serving Size
Milk, 1 cup
Cheese, 1 oz.
Yogurt, 1 cup
Buttermilk, 1 cup
Cottage cheese, 1 cup

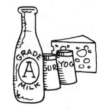

Minimum Daily Serving: 2

- Light and heavy foods
- 55-100 calories per exchange
- Milk exchange group

BREADS AND CEREALS provide B vitamins, iron, and chromium. Whole grains contain fiber, which helps prevent constipation. Whole grains are more nutritious than enriched products.

Serving Size
Bread, 1 slice
Rice, Noodles, Pasta, 1/2 cup as side dish,
    1 cup as main dish
Cereal, 1/2 cup cooked, 1 cup cold

Minimum Daily Serving: 4

- Light foods
- 70 calories per exchange
- Bread exchange group

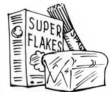

VITAMIN C-RICH FRUITS AND VEGETABLES. Vitamin C is needed to hold body cells together. It is also essential for strong blood vessel walls, proper immune response, and wound healing.

Serving Size
Orange juice, 1/2 cup
Grapefruit juice, 1/2 cup
Cantaloupe, 1/2
Grapefruit, 1/2
Orange, 1
Tomatoes, 2
Strawberries, 3/4 cup
Tangarines, 2
Papaya, 1/2
Bell pepper, 1/2

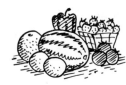

Minimum Daily Serving: 1

- Light foods
- 40 calories per exchange
- Choose one of your fruit exchanges from this list

DARK GREEN LEAFY VEGETABLES are excellent sources of Vitamin A and folic acid. Vitamin A helps keep your skin healthy, thereby protecting you against infection. It has also been shown to have a protective effect against certain types of cancers. Folic acid, a B vitamin, is necessary to form red blood cells and other body cells.

Serving Size
1 cup raw or 3/4 cup cooked:
    Asparagus
    Bok choy
    Broccoli
    Cabbage
    Swiss chard
    Spinach
    Greens
    Watercress
    Romain lettuce
    Red leaf lettuce

Minimum Daily Serving: 1

- Free foods
- 25 calories per exchange
- Vegetable exchange group

OTHER FRESH FRUITS AND VEGETABLES add other essential vitamins, minerals, and fiber to your diet. Those that are dark yellow in color contain Vitamin A.

Serving Size
Apple, 1
Banana, 1 small
Apricot, 2
Peach, 1
Pear, 1
Raisins, 2 Tbsp.
Dates, 2
Eggplant, 1/2 cup
Artichoke, 1

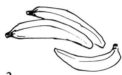

Minimum Daily Serving: 2

- Light foods
- Fruits are 40 calories per exchange
- Vegetables are 25 calories per exchange
- Fruit and vegetable exchange groups

If you consume nuts, nut butters, or seeds regularly, then there is no need for additional fats and oils in your diet. Remember, cooking with oil or butter COUNTS! So does dressing on your salad. Your body only needs 2 teaspoons of fat a day: safflower oil, soybean oil, sunflower oil.

5 CURRENT DIETARY ISSUES

People today generally do not have a problem getting the vitamins and minerals they need. The health hazards really come from EATING TOO MUCH:

- FAT
- SALT
- SUGAR
- WHITE FLOUR
- ALCOHOL

Eating "the American way" has been linked with the chronic degenerative diseases found so prevalently in our society: heart disease, cancer, hypertension, diabetes, and obesity. Even people who exercise regularly ARE NOT IMMUNE from these diseases, especially if their diet is made up of high-fat, refined foods.

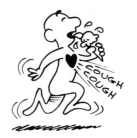

The overly processed foods we find on our grocery shelves, in restaurants, and in fast-food joints are a far cry from food in its natural state. They become ground, bleached, fried, preserved, hydrogenated, sweetened, and whatever else the manufacturer can think of. Is this food? Eating highly processed foods on a regular basis is not healthy. It results in a diet high in fat, high in salt, and low in fiber.

A diet high in FAT is correlated to:

- Heart disease (fat build-up in arteries)
- Breast cancer
- Colon cancer
- Obesity

A diet high in SALT is correlated with:

- High blood pressure
- Heart disease
- Strokes

A diet low in FIBER is correlated with:

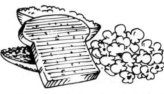

- Colon cancer
- Heart disease
- Obesity

- Diverticulosis (a disease of the large intestines in which outpouchings or pockets develop in the GI tract and can become inflamed and infected).

OBESITY is correlated with:

- Heart disease
- Cancer
- Diabetes

Rather than eating processed foods, concentrate on healthy foods. The positive side to this picture is that wholesome foods are:

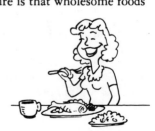

- Available
- Tasty
- Healthy
- Habit forming!

FIBER

Wholesome foods are also higher in FIBER. There has been a lot of publicity about fiber. It's supposed to be good for you, and easily obtained by eating bran cereals, bran muffins, and bran flakes. But what is fiber, and why is it best to maintain a high-fiber diet?

Fiber is roughage, residue, or bulk. It is only found in PLANT foods, since fiber consists of the cell walls that give plants their structure. Fiber is also found in the starchy parts of plants.

Humans cannot digest fiber. We do not have the proper

GI TRACT

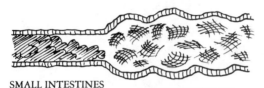

Residues, or fiber

SMALL INTESTINES

LARGE INTESTINES

enzymes to break down plant cell walls. Thus, fiber is what is left over after digestion takes place.

- Fiber helps maintain the health of your GI tract
- Fiber aids in controlling serum cholestrol levels
- Fiber helps regulate blood sugar levels
- Fiber helps fill you "up," not "out"

It is best to get your fiber requirement from whole foods, such as whole wheat flour, brown rice, bulgur wheat, and oatmeal. Adding BRAN to everything is NOT a good idea. Too much bran

GI TRACT

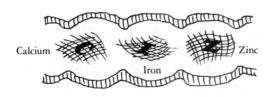

Calcium   Iron   Zinc

often leaches minerals from your system, such as iron and calcium. Therefore, bran can aggravate anemia or osteoporosis. Stick with whole foods instead of refined bran to keep your GI tract healthy and functioning properly.

Lean Toward High-Fiber Foods

Whole wheat bread
Oatmeal
Shredded wheat
Puffed wheat
Brown rice
Corn tortillas
Baked Potatoes
Rye crackers
Whole wheat noodles
Kidney beans
Lima beans
Pinto beans
White beans
Popcorn
Whole wheat bagels

Whole grain muffins
Whole grain pancakes, waffles
Bulgur
Berries
Pears
Oranges
Apples
Broccoli
Brussels sprouts
Carrots
Corn
Eggplant
Peas
Spinach
Winter squash

Use fresh fruit and vegetables instead of canned or frozen, whenever possible. They are generally higher in nutritional value and lower in sodium.

Low-Fiber Foods

White bread
Cream of wheat
Corn flakes
Puffed rice
White rice
Flour tortillas
French fries
Saltine crackers
Cookies

Meat
Fish
Poultry
Eggs
Sugar
Corn chips
Onion bagels
White four muffins
Bisquick pancakes/waffles

Pastries	White rice
White noodles	Fruit juice
Cheese	Fruit drinks
Yogurt	Vegetable Juices

CEREALS

Cereal is a common, often daily, food choice for breakfast. Thus, cereal can be a major source of good or bad nutrition. Start your day out RIGHT by choosing a recommended whole-grain cereal!

RECOMMENDED CEREALS are naturally high in fiber. Whole grains also contain chromium, a trace mineral that is **not** found in white, enriched cereals. People who eat chromium-rich diets may be protecting

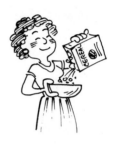

themselves from heart disease. Studies show that chromium-deficient diets speed up the process of fat build-up in the walls of the arteries.

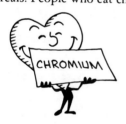

OK CEREALS are those that are:

- whole grain but contain too much added fat or sugar
- NOT whole grain but are not loaded with fat or sugar. They are missing fiber, chromium, and some B vitamins.

NOT RECOMMENDED CEREALS are either

- full of sugar or fat and not whole grain or
- over fortified with too many vitamins or minerals.

RECOMMENDED CEREALS

Whole Grain, Non-Commercial

Barley
Brown rice
Buckwheat
Cornmeal (whole)
Millet
Mixtures (4 grain,

9 grain)
Oats
Rye
Wheatberries
Wheat (cracked,
   bulgur)

Commercial Whole-grain, with

14% or Less Sugar
Instant Ralston
Nutri-Grain Cereal
Roman Meal
Rolled Oats
   (old-fashioned)
Skinner's Raisin Bran
Quaker Oat Bran
Wheatena
Zoom
Alpen

Back to Nature
Familia No
   Sugar Cereal
Grapenuts
Grapenut Flakes
Puffed Wheat
Shreaded Wheat
Wheat Chex
Wheaties
Wheetabix

OK CEREALS

Not Whole Grain:

Alber's Quick Grit
Cream of Rice
Cream of Wheat
Hominy grits

Wheat Hearts
Malt-o-Meal
Maypo
Oats, instant

Whole Grain, High in Fat or Sugar

BucWheats
C.W. Post

Fruit and Fiber
40% Bran Flakes

Familia   Granola
Fortified Oak Flakes

NOT Whole Grain

Life   Corn Chex
Special K   Cornflakes
All Bran   Cracklin' Bran
Bran Chex   Kix
Bran cereals   Puffed Rice
Cheerios, Toasty O's   Rice Chex
Cinnamon Life   Rice Krispies
Corn Bran   Team

NOT RECOMMENDED

High in Sugar or Over Fortified

Apple Jacks   Snack Pak
Cap'n Crunch   Sugar Frosted Flakes
Fruit Loops   Sugar Smacks
Golden Grahams   Trix
Honeycombs   Kellogg's Concentrate
Honey Nut Cheerios   Most
Kellogg's and Post's   Product 19
  Raisin Bran   Total
Oats, instant, flavored

FAT, SALT, AND SUGAR

The lists that follow tell you which foods you should emphasize or de-emphasize in your diet. A summary of the KEY reasons for making these

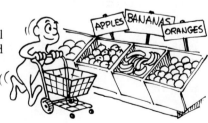

dietary changes precedes each list. Look over the foods carefully and find out which ones you ENJOY that happen to be good for you, too!

FAT

- Fats are artery blockers.

- Use as little fat in your diet as possible—that includes both animal and vegetable fats.

- Do NOT use fat substitutes— if you are going to eat a high-fat food, then eat a SMALL portion, and cut back to a **very** *low-fat* diet for the next few days. Fat substitutes generally do not promote proper nour- ishment at the cellular level.

- Use herbs and spices and VEGETABLES to flavor your food— NOT butter, margarine, sour cream, or oil.

Lean Away from High-Fat foods

Oil
Butter or margarine
Mayonnaise
Nondairy products
Sour cream
Cream
Half and half
Bacon
Lamb
Pork
Beef

Cheese
Luncheon Meats
Ice cream
Palm oil
Coconut
Whole milk
Gravy
Cream sauces
Cream soups
Doughuts

Lean Toward Low-Fat Foods

Chicken (no skin)
Turkey
Fish
Shellfish
Beans
Whole grains
Fresh fruit
Fresh vegetables
Corn tortillas

Brown rice
Oatmeal
Corn
Peas
Whole wheat noodles
Whole-grain crackers
Cottage cheese
Lowfat, nonfat yogurt
Buttermilk

THE PERCENTAGE OF FAT CALORIES IN YOUR FOOD

Over 50% Fat (Very High Fat)

Avocados
Coconut
Olives
Snack chips
Butter
Cream & sour cream
Cream cheese
Nondairy creamer
Hard cheeses
Nuts
Seeds
Tuna in oil
Eggs
Luncheon meats

Sausage
Spare ribs
Hot dogs
Salami
Pizza
Fried Chicken
Pork-loin, Boston butt
Beef, partially trimmed
Lamb, partially trimmed
Canadian bacon
Bacon
Ice cream
Clam chowder-white

30-50% Fat (High Fat)

French fries
Hash browns
Granola cereals

Ham
Fish sticks
Frozen dinners

Taco shells
Snack crackers
Whole milk
Chicken with skin
Turkey with skin
Beef, completely
  trimmed
Lamb, completely
  trimmed

Egg rolls
Taco
Cream soups
Cake
Pie
Candy Bars

15-30% Fat (Medium Fat)

Corn bread
Flour tortillas
Plain crackers
Buttermilk
Low fat cottage cheese
Fresh tuna
Bass
Clams

Crab
Oysters
Chicken, without skin
Turkey, without skin
Beef, round,
    completely trimmed
Veal, loin, round or
    shoulder, completely trimmed

Less than 15% Fat (Low Fat)

Fruits
Vegetables
Barley
Corn
Rice
Breads
Corn tortillas
Pasta
Pop corn
Rye crackers
Nonfat milk
Dried beans & peas
Waterchestnuts
Cod
Haddock

Halibut
Seabass
Sole
Tuna in water
Scallops
Shrimp
Squid
Egg whites
Spaghetti with tomato-
    mushroom sauce
Spices
Horseradish
Tabasco sauce
Vinegar
Broth

SALT

Salt intake is correlated with HIGH BLOOD PRESSURE. High blood pressure can be very harmful due to the:

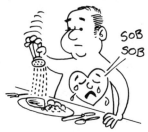

- increased work load on the heart, and
- damage to the arteries from the excessive pressure.

Lean Away from Foods High in Salt

Canned foods	V-8 juice
Frozen dinners	Luncheon meats
Cottage cheese	Hot dogs
Chips	Bacon
Salted nuts	Corned beef
Soy sauce	Parmesan cheese
Bouillon	Roquefort cheese
Instant hot cereal	American cheese
Olives	Frozen peas
Pickles	Corn flakes
Sauerkraut	Cheerios
Tomato juice	Special K

Lean Toward Foods Low in Salt

Herbs	Whole wheat flour
Garlic (Fresh or	Unsalted crackers
powdered)	Unsalted popcorn
Onion	Unsalted nuts
Tabasco sauce	Fresh fruit

Vinegar
Brown rice
Oatmeal (old-fashioned)
Whole-grain noodles
Corn tortillas
Puffed wheat
Shredded wheat

Fresh meats
Beans
Ricotta cheese
Most mineral waters
Tea
Coffee

Lean Toward Foods High in Potassium

Studies reveal that potassium helps to prevent hypertension (high blood pressure).

Cantaloupe
Bananas
Potatoes
Oranges
Grapefruit

Fresh tomatoes
Yellow squash
Spinach
Papaya
Beans

SUGAR

The average American eats more than 125 pounds of sugar a year. This seems like an amazingly high figure considering that sugar:

- Has NO nutritional benefits.
- Contributes to cavities.
- May elevate blood fat levels, which is a risk factor for heart disease.
- May contribute to the onset of diabetes in predisposed people.

The following list shows you **how** so much sugar can be consumed so easily—most of it is hidden in the foods you eat. The next time you put sugar in your cup of tea, figure out how much sugar is in the pastry you're eating with it!

Foods	Portion Size	Sugar Content (tsp.)
Bread/Cereals		
Whole wheat bread	1	1/4-1/2
Hot dog/hamburger bun	1	3
Dairy Products		
Ice cream	1/2 cup	4
Eggnog	8 oz.	4-1/2
Chocolate milk	5 oz.	6
Sherbet	1/2 cup	9
Beverages		
Cola drinks	12 oz.	9
Ginger ale	12 oz.	7
7-up	12 oz.	9
Desserts		
Apple pie	1 slice	7
Berry pie	1 slice	10
Cherry pie	1 slice	10
Lemon pie	1 slice	7
Peach pie	1 slice	7
Pumpkin pie	1 slice	5
Rhubarb pie	1 slice	4
Raisin pie	1 slice	13
Chocolate pudding	1/2 cup	4
French pastry	1 (4 oz.)	5
Chocolate sauce	1 Tbsp.	3-1/2
Hershey bar	1-1/2 oz.	2-1/2
Fudge	1 oz.	4-1/2
Hard candy	1 oz.	5

Foods	Portion Size	Sugar Content (tsp.)
Chocolate cake, iced	1 slice	10
Coffee cake	1 slice (4 oz.)	4½
Angel food cake	1 slice (4 oz.)	7
Pound cake	1 slice	5
Sugar cookie	1	2
Fig newton	1	5
Doughnut, glazed	1	6

Cereals	Sugar (%)
Shredded wheat	1
Cheerios	1.3
Grapenuts Flakes	3.3
Wheaties	4.4
Grapenuts	6.6
Corn flakes	7.8
BucWheats	13.6
Raisin Bran	13.6
Life	14
All Bran	20
Bran Buds	30
Frosted Flakes	44
Trix	46
King Vitamin	58
Sugar Smacks	61
Sugar Orange Crisp	68

ALCOHOL

Some people think that if they eat a nutritious diet, they don't have to worry about "a few drinks" every night before dinner. This is far from the truth. The following tells you why alcohol is hazardous to your health:

- People who drink a lot of alcohol are more likely to develop high blood pressure.

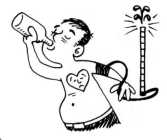

- Alcohol is toxic to the heart muscle; two drinks may produce impairment of heart muscle function.

- Alcohol in large dosages often produces irregular heart beats.

- Alcohol damages the liver.

- Alcohol often contributes to increased levels of blood fats (triglycerides and cholesterol).

- Alcohol raises the "wrong type" of HDL-cholesterol.

- Alcohol stimulates the release of insulin, a hormone that lowers your blood sugar level. Thus, you may experience symptoms of hypoglycemia: headache, shakiness, dizziness, and irritability.

- Alcohol uses up the B vitamins niacin and thiamin, making them unavailable for other essential functions.

- Alcohol interferes with the absorption of folacin and vitamin B^{12}.

- Alcohol increases urine output. Along with fluid, such minerals as magnesium, potassium, and zinc are also leached from your system.

Drink only 2 drinks per day, MAXIMUM. Better yet, save alcoholic consumption for a special occasion, such as wine with a candle-light dinner.

6 TIPS FOR DINING OUT AND DINING IN

Lots of people eat healthy foods at home, but "blow it" when they dine out. The problem is that many people go out to eat on a fairly regular basis. People are busy, tired, or don't feel like cooking. They may not even have much in the refrigerator—no time to grocery shop! By eating out frequently many people blow their healthy diet.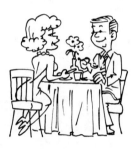

However, there's hope! You can eat out and still have a healthy, enjoyable meal. Here are some TIPS to help you maintain your new life-style of STAYING IN SHAPE. Read through the list and see which ideas will work for you.

- Frequent restaurants with salad bars or that serve generous salads. Eat lots of salad; this will make you less hungry for those high-fat foods.

- Go EASY on the salad dressing—1 to 2 tablespoons is enough. Help to control the portion by serving or ordering your salad dressing ON THE SIDE.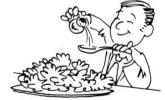

- Order salads instead of soups for dinner—soups are usually loaded with salt or fat. Remember: salad dressing on the side, PLEASE!

- Order "fancy" dishes with the sauce on the side. Use PORTION CONTROL!

- Stay away from cheese and cheese sauces. Instead, order tomato, garlic, wine, or herb sauces.

- Order food baked, broiled, or barbequed—**not fried**. Fried fish is often higher in fat than beef!

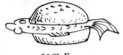

51% Fat

45% Fat

- Order chicken, fish, shellfish, turkey, veal, or vegetarian dishes. A serving size should be approximately the size of a chicken breast—or the palm of your hand.

- Order a plain baked potato, then add your own sour cream or butter—and a little dab will do it (1 to 2 teaspoons butter or 2 to 3 teaspoons sour cream)!

- When you order toast/bread, order it without butter, then add your own so you can see how little you really need.

- Order fresh fruit for dessert (papaya with lime, fresh strawberries, baked apple, cantaloupe).

- Control the amount of alcohol you consume. Order

    mineral water with lime
    Virgin Mary (spicy tomato juice)
    orange juice
    Half wine and half mineral water
    light beer
    light wine

There are two eating strategies. Choose the one that works best for you:

- Eat lots of light, healthy foods—salad, vegetables, potato (a

40

dab of butter). Eat FEWER fatty foods; leave high-fat foods until last, so that you are LESS HUNGRY and can use PORTION CONTROL. Or

■ Eat your favorite dish first—SLOWLY. STOP eating when you've had enough, rather than cleaning your plate.

■ SPEAK OUT, BE ASSER-
TIVE: Tell the waiter/wait-
ress you are watching your
fat intake. Are there any
special dishes he/she or
the cook might suggest.

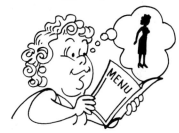

■ GIVE YOURSELF A PEP
TALK BEFORE ORDER-
ING: What is really important to me? Taste or a
trim, healthy body?

The best dining-out
tip is: Choose your res-
taurant carefully. It is
easier to order low-fat
foods at a seafood res-
taurant than at a Mexi-
can restaurant. PLAN
AHEAD.

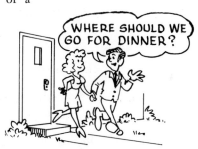

MENU IDEAS

Barbequed salmon, halibut

Seafood brochette

Scallops on a skewer

Baked scallops

Lobster tails with lemon

Mahi mahi

Cracked crab with hot sauce

Crab Louie (dressing on the side)

Alaskan king crab legs

Filet of sole (in a wine sauce)

Broiled swordfish

Veal piccata

Enchilada verde

Chicken teriyaki

Lemon chicken

Chicken cacciatori

Snow peas with chicken

Chef's salad (hold the ham & cheese;
more turkey, please!)

Egg flower soup

Spaghetti with clam sauce

Spaghetti with mushroom sauce

COOKING TIPS

At home, try using some of these cooking ideas—they will help lower the fat and salt in your diet. Experiment on your own, and go crazy with spices, mushrooms, green onions, red and green bell peppers, and tomatoes. It's important to realize that you can eat wonderful, flavorful foods without all that fat, sugar, and salt!

- Bake, broil, boil, steam, barbeque, or microwave foods—don't fry them!

- Use a rack when roasting meat so that it does not sit in the drippings.

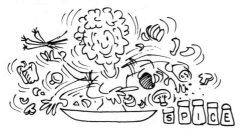

- Season vegetables with spices, lemon juice or peel, wine, green onions, parsley, watercress, red onions, mushrooms, peppers, or garlic.

- Saute vegetables in wine, chicken broth, or tomato juice.

- Serve fresh fruit for dessert; bake it in orange juice; top with fresh berries, a dab of ricotta cheese, slivered almonds, raisins.

- Wrap fish fillets in foil with a small amount of wine, onions, and tomatoes. There is no need for butter or oil.

- Bake turkey stuffing separately, using fat-free broth for flavor. Stuffing absorbs a lot of fat while baking the bird.

- Poach fish fillets in a stock mixture of clam juice and wine. Add herbs and reduce stock by half. Pour over cooked fillets.

- Avoid breading or flouring meat before browning, since the breading absorbs the meat fats.

- Use a **non-stick** pan, and use as little oil as possible while cooking.

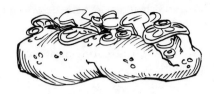

- Cover baked potatoes with lightly cooked tomatoes, mushrooms, and green onions.

- Use buttermilk, cottage cheese, ricotta, or yogurt as a base for salad dressings.

- Mix yogurt and apple juice as a topping for a fresh salad.

- Marinate chicken in orange juice, fresh ginger, and garlic. Baste it with this sauce while broiling.

- Make your food look attractive. Use sprigs of parsley, chopped green onions or fruit slices. Serve your meal on china dishes one night, and on other dishes the next night. It'll help make meal time a very enjoyable experience.

7 PHYSICAL ACTIVITY

Getting in shape means more than eating properly. It also means exercising regularly. People need to exercise to maintain their lean body tissue and lose their body fat. That is, KEEP ON THE GO!

EXERCISE

Keeping on the go is a healthy habit. People who MOVE their bodies experience the following joys:

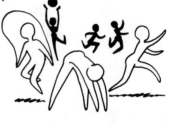

- They have fun.

- Their bodies get firm.

- They use up more calories.

- Their appetite diminishes.

- They feel great.

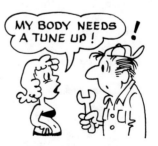

Exercisers experience even MORE BENEFITS than those listed above—such as CARDIOVASCULAR FIT-NESS. Exercising is a "tune up" for your heart, lungs, muscles, and blood vessels. An exerciser will have:

- Better circulation (tiny blood vessels open up to receive nourishment).

45

- A more efficient heart (your heart muscle gets bigger).

- More red blood cells (these cells carry oxygen to all your tissues).

- Lower blood pressure (this is the case for most people who exercise regularly).

- Healthier blood fats (fewer triglycerides and more HDL cholesterol—a "good guy" cholesterol that removes fat from your artery walls. There are about six different types of HDL cholesterol. Some are more beneficial than others.)

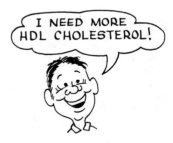

- Lower resting pulse rate (your heart is not working as hard as it used to, and a better job is being done).

- More muscle and less fat.

- Stronger bones (exercise promotes bone mineralization).

The best kind of exercise is AEROBIC, because it does all the **wonderful** things mentioned above. Aerobic activities do **more** than burn calories; they promote cardiovascular fitness.

Aerobic exercise simply means that the activity:

- Uses large muscle groups.

- Is continuous and rhythmic (not stop and go).

- Lasts at least 15 to 20 minutes or more.

- Is performed at least every other day (4 times per week).

When engaging in aerobic activity your body is utilizing

OXYGEN, and therefore producing lots of energy. Examples of aerobic exercise include the following activities:

- Walking briskly
- Jogging/running
- Swimming laps
- Ice skating
- Cycling
- Rowing
- Roller skating
- Skiing (especially cross-country)
- Aerobic dance
- Basketball
- Racquet ball*
- Tennis (singles).*

*These activities must last 45 to 60 minutes for cardivascular conditioning.

GETTING STARTED

If you're over thirty-five, or if you have any health concerns (high blood pressure, diabetes, heart disease), check *with your doctor* before starting an exercise program.

People who haven't exercised for a while may want to start off with a BRISK WALKING PROGRAM. Walking is great for people of all ages, and is excellent for general well being—mentally and physically.

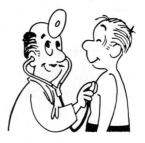

- Start your walking program gradually.

- Try walking slowly for a few minutes, then pick up your pace.

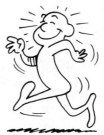

- Be able to TALK at all times during your exercise bout. If you can't talk, then you're exercising too fast.

- Set an exercise TIME for yourself. For example, you may want to start your program by walking 15 minutes, 3 times a week.

As your level of fitness increases, you'll want to pick up your pace, or walk for a longer period of time. You'll know when to make this change because you won't be tired or "worn out" after your work out!

After a while (anywhere from one to six months), you MAY want to start jogging. However, you may also want to remain a walker or engage in another form of exercise from the list on the previous page. Either way, many forms of exercise are fine for staying in shape. Keep in mind that cardiovascular fitness will occur FASTER with jogging than brisk walking. Also, some people find jogging more enjoyable than brisk walking.

If you choose to move on from a walking program to a more vigorous activity, be sure to start out gradually. You don't want sore muscles! For a jogging program, begin by walking briskly for a while, and then start jogging. Keep going until you feel tired. Then, start walking BRISKLY again until you catch your breath. Once again, pick up your pace and jog for a block or two. After a few weeks, you'll be jogging more and more, and walking less and less.

While jogging, cycling, swimming or engaging in any aerobic activity you will establish a pace that is comfortable for you. It is YOUR RHYTHM. Generally speaking, that pace will fall within your "TARGET ZONE." Your target zone is the heart beat count during exercise that is MOST BENEFICIAL for cardiovascular fitness.

- When your heart beats faster than the target zone recommends, you are adding stress on your system with little improvement in fitness.

- When your heart is beating slower than the target zone range, you are not conditioning your cardiovascular system in an optimal manner.

- Heartbeats and pulse rates will be the same. Usually it is easier to measure your pulse rate than to count your heart beats.

■ To determine your particular TARGET ZONE, use one of the following methods:

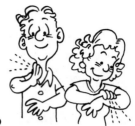

TARGET ZONES FOR CARDIOVASCULAR TRAINING

Method One

Chart for Target Heart Rates

Age	Heart Rate for 1 Minute	Heart Rate for 10 Seconds
20	140-170	23-28
25	137-166	23-28
30	133-162	22-27
35	130-157	22-26
40	126-153	21-26
45	125-149	21-25
50	119-145	20-24
55	116-140	19-23
60	112-136	19-23
65	109-132	18-22
70	105-128	18-21

METHOD TWO

Subtract your age from 220. Go for a target rate that is 70 to 85 percent of that figure. The target zone is really a RANGE instead of a specific number.

ON TARGET?

After you've been jogging for at least 3 minutes, STOP. Take your pulse at your wrist or at your neck. Check it for 10 seconds.

Are you in your TARGET ZONE for your age? If your heart is beating too fast, SLOW DOWN; you're over-doing it.

If your heart is not beating as fast as it should be, PICK UP YOUR PACE and check again. You need to work a little harder to get the conditioning effect you want. You want a GOOD tune-up!

KEEPING IN SHAPE

The rules for keeping in shape are to:

- Exercise 4 to 6 times a week.

- Exercise 20 to 30 minutes or more at a time.

- Exercise within your target zone for cardiovascular benefits.

Here are some other guidelines:

- Do some warm-up exercises before you work out. Be sure to start slowly for the first few minutes.

- DON'T come to a complete stop when you're done with your workout. Instead, end it with a brisk walk for about 5 minutes. Then, stretch again SLOWLY. After exercising, your blood is mainly in your "working" muscles. Your heart has to work extra hard to properly redistribute the blood in your muscles to other areas of your body. By walking after your workout, your muscles help **pump** the blood back into your circulatory system, making it easier on your heart.

- Wear proper clothes— no plastic attire—and proper shoes. If you choose to run, proper running shoes with good cushion are especially important.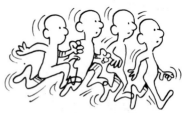

- Don't exercise if you're not feeling well.

- Beware—you may become HOOKED on exercise! It's wonderful.

8 CHANGE

It's important to know **what** is healthy to eat and **what** exercises to perform for cardiovascular fitness. It is also essential TO GET STARTED!

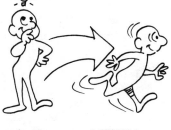

Knowledge has to be moved from the intellectual realm to practical application, or it's all for naught. One cannot get in shape by simply knowing the rules. It means ACTION.

This chapter discusses the issue of CHANGING, and maintaining that change. It includes a step-by-step procedure to help you implement your new knowledge. Read through the list and then write down one or two goals for yourself. This is a COMMITMENT to yourself, stating what you're willing and able to do. Start out slowly, and keep progressing forward. Before you know it, you'll be hooked on healthy habits. Enjoy!!

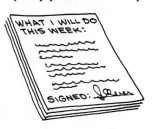

HOW TO CHANGE

Getting Started!

Step 1: DECIDE TO CHANGE

- You must decide for yourself that you want to change. Are YOU ready to do something about your habits?

Step 2: IDENTIFY THE PROBLEM

- Do you exercise infrequently?

- Do you eat too much cheese?

- Do you drink too much alcohol?

Step 3: DEVELOP A LIST OF ALTERNATIVES

Determine what habits you want to change, and what you'll do instead. Decide on a change you are WILLING to make. Your goal must be ATTAINABLE. Build success into your plans. For example, you can

- Drink nonfat milk instead of whole milk.

- Eat chicken instead of beef.

- Substitute 2 teaspoons butter for 2 tablespoons butter.

- Try tuna instead of cheese.

- Have fresh fruit for dessert instead of cake.

- Jog 3 times each week for 15 minutes.

Step 4: DO ONE OR MORE OF THESE ALTERNATIVES:

- Start walking briskly to work.

- Have fresh fruit in your refrigerator.

- Keep cookies out of the house.

Step 5: MONITOR YOUR PROGRESS

- How are you doing? Give your new habits a chance to work. Later, you might want to try other alternatives.

- Go back to Step 3 if you're having some difficulties.

Step 6: REALIZE THAT BIG CHANGES HAPPEN IN SMALL STEPS

- Small changes and tiny steps are SUCCESSES! People often write off small but important steps.

- Set one or two WEEKLY goals. Accomplish your new habits for only one week at a time. NOTE: It is important to outline a TIME FRAME for each goal.

Step 7: GIVE YOURSELF LOTS OF POSITIVE SELF-TALK

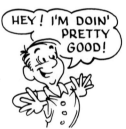

- If you don't make your goal, that's OK. Nobody is perfect. Change is NOT a smooth process. There are always stalls, plateaus, barriers and problems!

- Start fresh the next day—you'll make it this time!

- Give yourself ENCOURAGING words. They spur you on to success. DON'T discourage yourself.

- Concentrate on what you do right.

MAINTAINING CHANGE

Keep Going

Once you have made some healthy habit changes, you will want to keep them. An easy way to make sure you stay on track is by keeping a CHECKLIST—a mental and physical one. Periodically review your checklist of habits to keep. If you aren't following it, find your problem area and work on IMPROVING IT. Choose ONE area at a time, so you won't overwhelm yourself. Being overwhelmed leads to discouragement— the BIGGEST ENEMY of change. Keep a positive outlook and be persistent. Tell yourself YOU are on TOP of the situation, the situation is NOT on top of you. Then, start eating lightly and exercising regularly again.

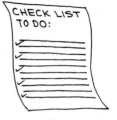

Here are some TIPS on how to maintain your new life-style:

- ***Weigh yourself once a week.*** If you have gained some weight, plan to lose it immediately. Set a goal: lose 1 to 2 pounds each week, eating FREE and LIGHT foods only. USE A REWARD: When you lose the weight, buy yourself something special or spend time with a special friend or do something else nice for yourself.

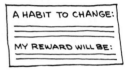

- ***Check your habits each week.*** If you are backsliding, pick ONE HABIT to change each week. LIST an alternative habit, and then DO it.

CHECKLIST OF GOOD HABITS:

- Do aerobic exercises 4 to 5 times a week, such as swimming, jogging, brisk walking, cycling, or aerobic dancing.

- Eat mainly free and light foods, such as fruit, vegetables, and other light foods; and stay away from foods that are high in sugar, fat, and salt.

- Eat small or average amounts, such as one piece of chicken, rather than two; one sandwich rather than two.

- Keep high-fat, high-sugar foods out of the house. Make an UN-shopping list and don't bring home sweets.

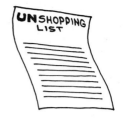

- Use a "thin" eating style: eat slowly and relax before eating.

- Drinking alcohol in moderation. Drink alcohol on special occasions, NOT as a regular habit.

- Have a healthy eating environment. Have food only in the kitchen, leaving it out of sight to discourage nibbling. Have LOTS of free and light food available.

- Eat when hungry, stopping when you are just **satisfied**. Satisfied does not mean full, and definitely not stuffed.

- Feel hunger pangs. Try to feel hungry for a couple of hours each day.

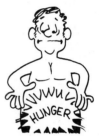

- Be active. Spend time moving around instead of sitting.

- Deal consciously with special occasions. Decide on a food strategy, such as eating lots of free and light foods, saying "no thanks," and giving yourself encouraging words.

- Treat yourself well. Think of your good qualities, about what you do well, instead of giving yourself discouraging words.

- Maintain a supportive environment. Be around friends who encourage healthy eating habits and regular exercise. Find a buddy to jog with.

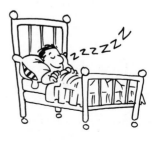

- Get plenty of rest. When you are tired, you're more apt to overeat.

9 DOING IT

Now you know about the EXCHANGE SYSTEM and the facts concerning PROCESSED FOODS. You also know the importance of regular, AEROBIC EXERCISE and how to get started. In this chapter you'll learn how to use this knowledge on a day-to-day basis in order to get IN SHAPE.

The following is an example of someone who is:

- Developing an exchange strategy to lose weight.

- Plugging exchanges into menu plans.

- Keeping an exercise log.

- Writing a short, personal diary.

MY EXCHANGE STRATEGY

Food	Number of Exchange	Calories
Starches	4	280
Vegetables	From free foods list ONLY	
Fruit	3	120
Milk	2	180
Protein (lean and medium fat ONLY)	5	332.5
Fats	2	90
TOTAL		1002.5

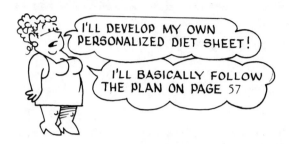

"I'll write myself a list of menus* so I won't have to think about it the rest of the week. I'll just simply follow my personalized diet sheet!"

"I'll keep an exercise log. That'll keep me exercising regularly, and I'll be able to follow my progress. I'll also write down my thoughts and see how my outlook develops concerning my SHAPING UP Program."

*For a diet with less variety, but also less time and thought, turn to page 71 .

Day 1

Breakfast	Exchange
1 cup shredded wheat	1 bread
1 cup nonfat milk	1 milk
1 small banana	1 fruit
Coffee	0

I HAVE TWO MORE FRUITS LEFT.

Morning Snack	
1 apple	1 fruit

Lunch	
Turkey sandwich:	
bread, 2 slices whole wheat	2 breads
2 oz. turkey	2 proteins
Tomato slices	0

Alfalfa sprouts	0
1 orange	1 fruit
1 glass nonfat milk	1 milk

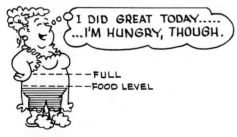

LET'S SEE, I'VE USED UP ALL MY FRUITS, BUT I HAVE A STARCH LEFT FOR DINNER.

Afternoon Snack

V-8 juice	0
2 raw carrots	0

Dinner

Barbequed chicken breast	3 proteins
1 red potato with	1 starch
1 tsp. butter	1 fat
Large salad with low-calorie dressing	0
Broccoli	0
1 tsp. butter	1 fat

Late Snack

Mineral water and lime
Cole slaw with low-calorie dressing

I DID GREAT TODAY..... ...I'M HUNGRY, THOUGH.

— FULL
— FOOD LEVEL

Exercise Log/Diary

I walked and jogged 10 minutes away from my front door step, then turned around, so that's 10 minutes back again—20 minutes

TOTAL. It felt good. Big changes happen in small steps.

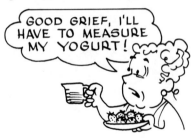

Day 2

Breakfast	Exchange
2/3 cup nonfat yogurt	1 milk
3/4 cup strawberries	1 fruit
1/2 English muffin with	1 starch
1 tsp. butter	1 fat
Tea	0

Morning Snack	
1 orange	1 fruit

Lunch	
Large salad with	0
2 oz. tuna and	2 proteins
1 Tbsp. dressing	2 fats
1 whole-grain roll (no butter)	2 starches

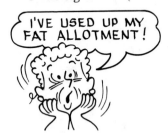

Afternoon Snack	
Glass of nonfat milk	1 milk

Dinner

3 oz. red snapper poached in wine, garlic, and spices	3 proteins
1/2 cup brown rice	1 starch
Zucchini and red peppers, lightly steamed	0

> WOW! I USUALLY HAVE SO MUCH MORE RICE THAN THIS. I WANT MORE!

Late Snack

1 pear	1 fruit

Exercise Log/Diary

I walked-jogged for *20 minutes* again today. It was easier to do than yesterday. Still felt like a cheeseburger and fries for dinner. I made myself fix a seafood dish and, hey, it wasn't too bad! In fact, I liked it.

Day 3

Breakfast	Exchange
2 eggs	2 proteins
1 slice oatmeal bread	1 starch
1/2 cup orange juice	1 fruit

Morning Snack

1 doughnut	165 calories
Coffee	0

> OH NO! I BLEW MY DIET. SOMEONE BROUGHT THESE TO WORK AND I COULDN'T RESIST THEM. I KNOW IF I EXERCISE FOR 30 MINUTES I'LL BURN UP THE CALORIES IN THIS LOUSY DOUGHNUT.

Lunch

Crab Sandwhich:	
2 slices bread	2 breads
2 oz. crab	2 proteins
2 tsp. mayonnaise	2 fats
Lettuce	0

Afternoon Snack

1 small banana	1 fruit

Dinner

Large salad:	
1/4 cup cottage cheese	1 protein
2/3 cup nonfat yogurt	1 milk
1 diced apple	1 fruit
Romaine lettuce	0

Late Snack

1 glass nonfat milk	1 milk

Day 4

Breakfast	Exchange
1 bran muffin (no butter)	2 starches
1 glass milk	1 milk
1/2 grapefruit	1 fruit
Coffee	0

Morning Snack

Handfull of red grapes	1 fruit

Lunch

Peanut-butter-banana sandwich:	
2 slices whole wheat bread	2 starches
4 tsp. peanut butter	2 fats
1/2 large banana, slice	1 fruit
1 glass nonfat milk	1 milk

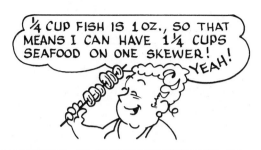

Dinner

BBQ seafood (5 oz.) brochette:	
Scallops, halibut, prawns	5 proteins
mushrooms, onions, bell	
pepper, cherry tomatoes	0
Large salad with free vegetables	
and low-calorie dressing	0

Exercise Log/Diary

I didn't have time to jog today, but I only need to exercise 3 to 4 times a week. I feel better when I get it in, though. I'll be sure to jog tomorrow. I'll get my bubdy to join me. It's more fun that way.

Day 5

Breakfast

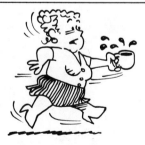

"No time to fix breakfast this morning. I grabbed a cup of coffee and ran out the door."

Lunch

Turkey sandwich:	
2 slices whole wheat bread	2 starches
3 oz. turkey	3 proteins
1 tsp. mayonnaise	1 fat
Lettuce	0

Tomato	0
1 orange	1 fruit
Handful of grapes	1 fruit
1 glass nonfat milk	1 milk

Afternoon Snack

8 almonds	1 fat
2 Tsp. raisins	1 fruit

Dinner

1 cup whole-grain pasta	2 starches
2 oz. lean beef in tomato and mushroom sauce	2 proteins
Spinach salad with fresh mushrooms and low-calorie dressing	0

Late Snack

1/2 cup low-fat yogurt	1 milk
1¼ cup raspberries	2 fruits

Exercise Log/Diary

I walked-jogged for *20 minutes*. I jogged more today and walked less. That felt good.

I rode my bicycle for *12 minutes* after my evening snack. I was going to eat my yogurt with FREE VEGETABLES, but I didn't feel like eating vegetables.

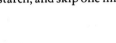

"I'm going out to dinner and I want a glass of wine. Let's see, I'll save up one starch, and skip one milk."

Day 6

Breakfast	Exchange
1/2 cup whole-grain roll	1 starch

2 tsp. peanut butter (old fashioned)	1 fat
1/2 cantaloupe	2 fruits
1 cup nonfat milk	1 milk

Lunch

Salad with free vegetables— carrots, zucchini, red peppers, mushrooms, tomatoes, red onions, romaine lettuce, jicama—and low-calorie dressing	0
1 apple	1 fruit
Coffee	0

Afternoon Snack

| Raw carrots | 0 |
| Mineral water and lime | 0 |

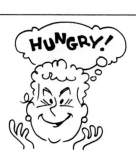

Dinner (out)

1 glass white wine	90 calories
5 oz. broiled halibut	5 proteins
1 Large baked potato with	2 starches
1 tsp. butter	1 fat
Large salad with 1/2 Tbsp. dressing	1 fat

Day 7

Breakfast

1 cup oatmeal	2 starches
2 Tbsp. raisins	1 fruit
8 almonds	1 fat

1 orange	1 fruit
1 cup nonfat milk	1 milk
Coffee	0

Lunch

1/2 cup cottage cheese	2 proteins
1 slice small banana	1 fruit
Mineral water and lemon	0

I'M FULL!

Afternoon Snack

| 3 cups popcorn (no fat added) | 1 starch |
| Diet soda | 0 |

Dinner

3/4 cup shrimp in	3 proteins
creole sauce (no fat)	0
1/2 cup brown rice	1 starch
String beans with mushrooms	0
1/2 cup ice cream	200 calories

Exercise Log/Diary

Jogged for *20 minutes.* I didn't walk at all this time! I did well on my diet today, except for dessert. That's OK, though, I'll just DEDUCT 1 STARCH and 2 FATS from tomorrow's diet. I can do it. Positive self-talk, that spurs me on to success!

Day 8

Breakfast	Exchange
1½ cup puffed wheat	1 starch
1 cup nonfat milk	1 milk
3/4 cup berries	1 fruit
Coffee	0

Morning Snack

V-8 juice	0

Lunch

1 slice bread	1 starch
2 oz. tuna, water packed	2 proteins
Sprouts	0
Tomatoes	0
Cucumbers	0
1 glass nonfat milk	1 milk

Afternoon Snack

1 peach	1 fruit

Dinner

3 oz. turkey (no gravy)	3 proteins
1/2 cup mashed potatoes	1 starch
Artichoke (no fat)	0
Spinach salad with	0
orange slices and	1 fruit
low-calorie dressing	0

Exercise Log/Diary

I jogged for *25 minutes* today. I'll do this for one week and try for 30 minutes next week.

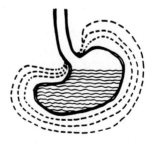

At the beginning of this diet, I got awfully hungry at times. When I finished a meal, I didn't FEEL finished. I still wanted MORE FOOD.

Now, I'm as full after my meals as I was when I ate BIG meals. Thank heavens! My stomach has adjusted, and it's so much easier.

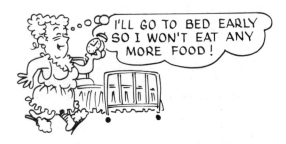

Day 9

Breakfast	Exchange
Two 5" oatmeal pancakes	70 calories each or 2 starches
1¼ cup raspberries,	2 fruits
1 cup nonfat milk	1 milk
Coffee	0

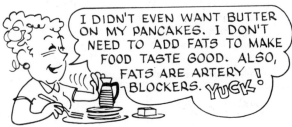

Lunch

Cole slaw:	
red cabbage, green cabbage,	
carrots, peppers with	0
Low-calorie dressing	0
1 cup cottage cheese	4 proteins
1 red apple	1 fruit

Afternoon Snack

Mineral water and lime	0

Dinner

1 cup vegetarian chili with	2 starches
1/2 oz. grated cheese	1 protein

1/2 cup low-fat yogurt	1 milk
Shredded lettuce, diced tomatoes,	
peppers, and green onions	0

Exercise Log/Diary

I jogged for *25 minutes* today. I tried to pick up my pace a bit.
I ate only 1/2 oz. cheese, since it is 100 calories per ounce. In my initial menu plan, I decided to eat ONLY LEAN and MEDIUM fat protein foods. So I made up for my "cheat" by eating only half a portion.

Day 10

Breakfast	Exchange
1 cup shredded wheat	1 starch
1 small banana	1 fruit
1 cup nonfat milk	1 milk
Coffee	0

Lunch

Cold pasta salad:	
1 cup whole wheat pasta shells	2 starches
1/2 cup shrimp	2 proteins
Green and red bell peppers,	
tomatoes, and green onions,	
with low-calorie dressing	0
1 apple	1 fruit
Tea	0

Dinner

Turkey enchiladas:	
3 oz. turkey	3 proteins
1 corn tortilla	1 starch
Enchilada sauce (no fat)	0
1/2 cup low-fat yogurt	1 milk

Late Snack

Baked apple with cinnamon	1 fruit
8 almonds	1 fat

I jogged for *30 minutes*. I didn't push myself, because I was in my TARGET ZONE. (I checked it after 3 minutes of jogging.)

I decided to LEAVE OUT the CHEESE on my enchilada. It tasted great without it! The yogurt alone was fine. Also, if I want to add calories to my diet, I'll add STARCH calories, since they DON'T contribute to heart disease. I know that people can be THIN and have CLOGGED ARTERIES.

Day 11

Breakfast

1 cup oatmeal	2 starches
2 slices toast	2 starches
1¼ cup fresh berries	2 fruits
1 cup nonfat milk	1 milk

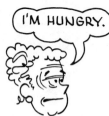

Lunch

Turkey sandwich:	
2 slices bread	2 starches
4 oz. turkey	4 proteins
1 apple	1 fruit
1 cup nonfat milk	1 milk

Afternoon Snack

8 almonds	1 fat
2 Tbsp. raisins	2 fruits

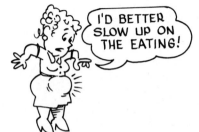

Dinner

Large salad with Low-calorie dressing	0

Exercise Log/Diary

I jogged harder today since I "blew" my diet . . . or did I? After adding up the calories, I only ate 1,065 calories today. That's great! Also, they were low-fat, high-fiber calories. ALL RIGHT! My fat cells love me, and so do my arteries.

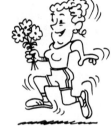

I'm beginning to PREFER to eat healthy foods. They taste great! Also, I feel good about myself when I eat this way.

Exercising regularly has really helped me lose weight. However, I like to exercise because I want to be MORE THAN THIN—I want to be FIT. Almost every time I jog, my mental attitude improves by 200 percent. It's great for boosting my spirits.

SIMPLIFIED WEIGHT-LOSS FOOD PLAN

Some people want a simple, hassle-free diet to follow. Therefore, I developed a SIMPLIFIED WEIGHT-LOSS FOOD PLAN for those who don't want to be bothered with menu planning, food preparation, or left-overs! Choose a menu for breakfast, lunch, and dinner. Vary them, so that you don't become bored with eating the same foods. It's IMPOR-TANT when you start out to meas-ure your food for portion control. Later you can eye-ball the proper amounts.

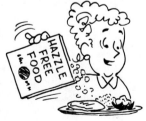

Breakfast

1 egg
1 slice whole wheat toast
  (**easy** on the butter or margarine)
1 piece fresh fruit
Coffee, tea, water, or nonfat milk

Menu #2:

1 cup dry cereal (sugarless variety)
  or 1/2 cup hot cereal
1 cup nonfat milk
1 piece fresh fruit
Coffee, tea, or water

Lunch

Menu #1:

Open-faced sandwich
  (*easy* on the fats: mayonnaise, butter, etc.)
One piece fresh fruit
Coffee, tea, water, or nonfat milk

Menu #2:

Fresh fruit, 1 to 2 pieces
1/2 to 1 cup low-fat cottage cheese
Coffee, tea, water

Menu #3:

Fresh fruit, 1 to 2 pieces
1/2 to 1 cup low-fat or nonfat plain yogurt
Coffee, tea, water

Menu #4:

Large salad* (containing one protein:
  chicken, seafood, or turkey)
1 small roll (preferably whole grain)
Coffee, tea, or water

Dinner

Menu #1:

    1 cup casserole (low in fat and cheese)
    Tossed green salad*
    Vegetables (no added fat)
    Coffee, tea, water

Menu #2:

    4 oz. or 1 cup chicken, fish, seafood, or lean meat
    Tossed green salad*
    Vegetables (no added fat)
    1/2 cup rice or 1 small potato or 1/2 cup pasta

*Have your dressing on the side, and add no more than *one* tablespoon to your salad.

Exercise Equivalents of Calories

In general, AEROBIC exercise utilizes 10 to 15 calories per minute and RECREATIONAL exercise utilizes 4 to 8 calories per minute.

MINUTES TO BURN OFF 100 CALORIES

Activity	Minutes
Run/jog	9
Climb stairs	10
Saw wood	10
Raquetball	10
Swim	10
Jump on trampoline	12
Soccer	13
Aerobic dance	15
Dig in garden	17
Cycle	18
Walk	20
Volleyball	20
Scrub floors	20

Note:
    Exercise can "burn up" the calories in high-fat foods. But what about your arteries? You don't want too much fat circulating in your blood stream. It can build up!

CONCLUSION

You're well on your way to BEING IN SHAPE. Enjoy the benefits of a firm, strong, healthy body—a cheerful, positive outlook on life. Slowly changing your life-style is worth every bit of your time and effort, because the payoffs are there. Indulge yourself in your newfound pleasures. It feels sooo good!

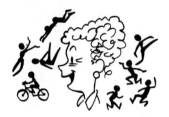

CALORIES IN FOOD

Beverages	Amount	Calories
Beer	12 oz.	150
Brandy	1 oz.	65
Gin	1½ oz.	130
Liquers	1 oz.	70-115
Rum	1½ oz.	130
Vodka	1½ oz.	130
Whiskey	1½ oz.	130
Lite beer	12 oz.	70-95
Red wine	4 oz.	100
White wine	4 oz.	95
Cola	12 oz.	145
Ginger ale	12 oz.	115
Root beer	12 oz.	150
Tonic water	8 oz.	72
Collins mix	8 oz.	112
Lemonade	8 oz.	100
Apple juice	8 oz.	120
Pineapple juice	8 oz.	150

Desserts		
Cheesecake	1 slice	450
Chocolate cake with icing	1 slice	235
Apple pie	1 slice	300
Pumpkin pie	1 slice	240
Pecan pie	1 slice	430
Danish pastry	1	275
Doughnut, glazed	1	165
Fig cookie	1	50
Gingersnap	1	30
Cookie, chocolate chip	1	90
Marshmallow	4	90

Candy	Amount	Calories
Life Saver	1	10
Lemon drop	1	15
Gum drops	10	50

Snack Foods

	Amount	Calories
Dry roasted peanuts	1/2 cup	425
Cashews	8	67
Saltine crackers	4 square	50
Corn chips	1/4 cup	60
Potato chips	5	60
Graham crackers	2 squares	50
Melba toast	1	15
Pretzels	10	8

Potatoes

	Amount	Calories
Au gratin	1/2 cup	180
French fries	10	215
Hash browns	1/2 cup	175
Mashed potatoes	1/2 cup	
milk added		70
milk and butter added		100
"Home fries"	1/2 cup	230

Main Dishes

	Amount	Calories
Macaroni and cheese	1/2 cup	215
Spaghetti and tomato sauce	3/4 cup	195
Pizza	1 slice	250

Side Dishes

	Amount	Calories
3-bean salad	1/2 cup	337
Cream of mushroom soup	1 cup	216
Chicken and rice soup	1 cup	48
Split pea soup	1 cup	130

Breads/Cereals	Amount	Calories
Muffin	1	150
Bagel	1	165
English muffin	1	140
Banana bread	1 slice	119
Pancake	4″ diam.	60
Waffle	1	210
French toast	1 slice	88
Granola	3/4 cup	375

Milk Products		
Hot cocoa	1 cup	240
Thick shake	12 oz.	430
Chocolate malt	8 oz.	500
Ice milk	1/2 cup	100
Ice cream	1/2 cup	175
Sherbet	1/2 cup	130
Frozen yogurt	6 oz.	150
Fruit flavored yogurt	1 cup	250

RECIPES

The following recipes are sumptuous and simple. They are also good for you! The recipes and menu ideas are to help you get started on your new life-style changes. This means eating less meat and more grains, legumes, and vegetables as a main dish. Therefore, you will find pancake and pasta recipes, instead of omelet and beef dishes. By eating this way, you will decrease your fat intake and increase your fiber consumption. Also, plant foods are loaded with vitamins and minerals.

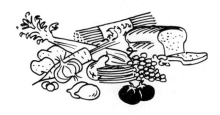

Breads

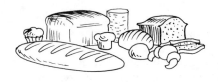

Cindy's Whole Wheat Bread
Makes 2 loaves.

This bread is excellent. If you grind your own wheat, it's even better!

2 packages yeast
1 cup warm water
1/3 cup honey
2 cups low-fat milk
1/4 cup 2 Tblsp. oil + 2 Tblsp. butter
1 Tblsp. salt
5 cups Stone-Buhr whole wheat flour
3 cups whole wheat pastry flour *or*
   Gold Medal whole wheat flour

Sprinkle yeast into water and add part of honey. Let sit 10 minutes. Combine remaining honey with milk, butter, oil, and salt. Heat until butter melts. Cool mixture until luke warm, then stir in yeast mix. Stir in all of the Stone-Buhr whole wheat flour and blend until smooth. Add rest of flour. Knead until smooth, for 10 minutes or so. Place dough in buttered pan aand cover with a towel. Let rise in a a warm place for 1 hour or until doubled. Punch down and knead dough a few times. Let it set another 10 minutes. Divide dough in half and knead each half. Shape into loaves and place in buttered 9x5x3" pans. Let rise until doubles (about 30 minutes). Bake at 400 for 40 minutes or until hollow when tapped.

Irish Soda Bread
Makes 1 loaf

I add chopped dried apricots, raisins, and walnuts to this recipe. Some people add caraway seeds, too.

2 cups whole wheat flour
3/4 tsp. baking soda
1/2 cup low-fat or nonfat plain yogurt
1/4 cup plus 2 Tblsp. water

Mix flour and baking soda. Mix yogurt and water and blend with flour mixture. Knead 5 minutes or less. Form into ball. Make three slits with a knife across dough. Brush with milk. Bake at 400° F for 35 to 40 minutes. Serve while warm. No need to spread with fat (butter or margarine), it tastes so good just plain.

Oatmeal Apple Muffins
Makes 12 muffins

1½ cup sour milk (1 cup skim milk + 1 Tblsp. vinegar)
2 cups rolled oats
1 cup whole wheat flour
1 tsp. baking soda
1 or 2 eggs
2 Tblsp. honey
1/2 cup raisins
2 apples, chopped
2 tsp. cinnamon
1 tsp. allspice

In a large bowl soak oats in sour milk overnight in the refrigerator or for 2 hours outside of refrigerator. After soaking add other ingredients and stir until well blended. Bake at 400°F for 20 minutes.

Michelle's Oatmeal Pancakes
Makes about 15 pancakes

Michelle is a jogger who has lost excess poundage lately. She is eating a low-fat, low-sugar diet. She often serves oatmeal pancakes for dinner, along with a large fresh-fruit salad.

1½ cups old-fashioned oatmeal
3/4 cup nonfat yogurt
1¼ cup nonfat milk
2 apples, diced
1 tsp. honey
1 tsp. baking soda
1/2 cup whole wheat flour
2 eggs
1/2 tsp. salt (optional)

Mix oats, yogurt, and milk in a bowl. Let stand for 5 minutes. Add the rest of the ingredients and mix. Using a 1/4 cup measure, scoop out batter onto a nonstick pan. Cook over a medium heat. Serve with a dollop of yogurt.

Cottage Cheese Pancakes
Serves 4

This is a high-protein pancake. There is no need to serve them with eggs, since there are enough in the batter. I put warm homemade applesauce on top of these pancakes.

1 cup whole wheat flour
1 tsp. baking powder
1 Tblsp. honey
4 eggs, well beaten
2 cups low-fat cottage cheese
1/4 cup skim milk

Mix the dry ingredients well. Add honey, eggs, and cottage cheese. Stir in the milk. Cook on a hot griddle until well browned on both sides.

Note: The batter is quite thick, but the pancakes are light and fluffy. For a thinner batter, increase the skim milk to 1/2 cup.

Anna's Pancakes
Makes about eighteen 4-inch cakes

Anna sneaks out to her kitchen early and prepares these wholesome pancakes for the morning joggers in the family. They're yummy with fresh-fruit purees.

2 cups whole wheat flour
1 tsp. soda
2 eggs, well beaten
2 cups buttermilk
2 Tblsp. oil
1 Tblsp. honey (optional)

Blend dry ingredients together into a bowl. Combine wet ingredients and add to dry ones, stirring only until flour is moistened. Drop by spoonfuls onto hot griddle.

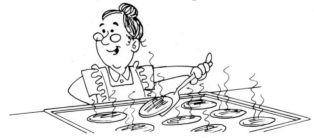

Pancake Toppings

Try these instead of syrup and butter. They are a delicious change, and they don't leave you with that heavy feeling.

Strawberry Puree
Serves 3.

3/4 cup sliced fresh strawberries
1 Tblsp. apple juice concentrate
1 tsp. honey

Place ingredients in a blender. Puree and pour into a serving dish. Serve over warm whole-grain pancakes.

Fruit and Yogurt Delight
Serves 2-3.

1/2 cup chopped dried fruit (I use peaches, apricots,
    and apples, but any fruit works)
2 Tblsp. apple juice concentrate
1/2 cup water
1/2 cup yogurt

Place fruit, 1 tablespoon apple juice concentrate, and water in a
saucepan. Cook over medium heat until fruit is plump and tender.
Mix fruit into yogurt along with 1 tablespoon apple juice
concentrate. Serve over warm whole-grain pancakes or waffles.

Fruit Sauce
Serves 2-3.

The following recipe is somewhat high in sugar. However,
because you can use this without butter or syrup, it is a good, tasty
alternative for a topping on pancakes or waffles.

1/3 cup ricotta cheese
2 Tblsp. raspberry jam
1 tsp. lemon juice
1/4 cup skim milk
1/2 tsp. vanilla
1 Tblsp. honey

Blend all ingredients. Serve on whole-grain pancakes.

Main Dishes

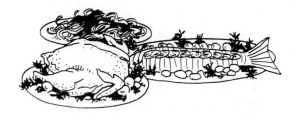

Snapper a la Rod
Serves 4.

This is an easy company dish that is not only good for you, but is fancy and delicious. Rod, my running buddy, makes this for special occasions.

2 Tblsp. olive oil
4 small red snapper fillets
2 fresh tomatoes, diced
1 cup fresh mushrooms, sliced
1/2 cup chopped onion
1/2 cup green pepper
1/3 cup dry white wine
1/4 cup chopped parsley
1 garlic clove, crushed
1/4 tsp. pepper
1/4 tsp. thyme, crushed
1 bay leaf

Heat oil in a skillet and lightly brown snapper in it. Add remaining ingredients. Bring to a boil, then simmer, covered, for about 10 mintues—until the fish just flakes when tested with a fork. Remove fish to a heated platter and keep warm in oven. Simmer liquid in pan to about 1/4 cup (about 5 minutes). Spoon over fish. Serve with brown rice and tossed green salad.

Sea Bass and Fennel
Serves 4.

1 Tblsp. oil
2 fennel roots
1/2 cup water
or 1/4 cup water and 1/4 cup chicken broth
2 lb. sea bass (or red snapper)

Lightly saute fennel in oil in a nonstick skillet. Add liquid. Cook 1/2 hour, adding more liquid if necessary. Add fish and poach in liquid. Cook until the fish flakes when tested with a fork, about 10 minutes. Remove to a warm platter and keep warm in oven. Boil liquid for 5 minutes to brown fennel. Serve fillets with fennel over them. Serve with cold pasta salad and crisp green salad.

Lemon Chicken
Serves 4.

This is a simple recipe, but very tasty. The lemon flavor permeates the chicken.

2½ lb. whole chicken
Salt and pepper to taste
2 lemons

Preheat oven to 350°F. Wash and dry the chicken. Season inside of bird with salt and pepper. Pierce lemons with a fork 20 times. Put into chicken cavity. Tie chicken legs together, sealing the cavity closed. Put chicken in pan, breast side down. Cook 15 minutes. Turn chicken over and cook 20 minutes longer. Turn up oven to 400°F and cook for another 20 minutes.

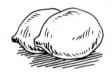

Ayn's Chicken
Serves 4.

This is one of my favorites. I garnish this dish with chopped green onions and slivered almonds.

For Marinade:
  2 tsp. oil
  2 tsp. tamari (soy sauce)
  Dash of fresh ground pepper
  4 chicken breast halves, boned and flattened to 1/2 inch
  Cornstarch or arrowroot

Combine first 3 ingredients and rub over chicken. Coat chicken lightly with cornstarch. Refrigerate at least 30 minutes.

For Sauce:
  2 Tblsp. tomato paste
  3/4 cup water
  2 tsp. honey
  2 Tblsp. lemon juice
  1 tsp. cornstarch dissolved in 2 tsp. water

Combine first 4 ingredients in sauce pan. Bring to a boil, stirring. Add dissolved cornstarch and stir till thickened. Set aside and keep warm.

For Chicken:
  2 tsp. oil
  2/3 cup bean sprouts
  2/3 cup snow peas
  2/3 cup water chestnuts
  1/2 large *red* bell pepper, sliced

Heat 1 tsp. of the oil in a nonstick pan. Cook chicken in the oil until golden brown. Drain and cut into 2/3-inch strips. Keep warm. Add the other tsp. of oil to pan, heat vegetables until crisp and tender, about 5 minutes. Transfer to heated platter. Top with chicken and spoon sauce over it. Enjoy!

Chicken-Bulgur Pilaf
Serves 4.

This is a fun dish to serve guests. Place condiments in the center of the table and let people pile on their own toppings.

2 Tblsp. oil
4 chicken breasts, skinned
2 medium onions, sliced
2 cloves garlic, chopped
1½ Tblsp. curry powder
Salt to taste (about 1/2 tsp.)
1 cup bulgur
1 can (14 oz.) chicken broth
1/2 tsp. cinnamon
Condiments

Brown chicken in oil in a non-stick pan. Set chicken aside. Heat onion, garlic, curry powder, salt, and bulgur in same skillet, stirring about 5 minutes. Add broth and cinnamon. Bring to a boil, add chicken, reduce heat, cover, and simmer until chicken is tender, 25 to 35 minutes. Serve with bowls of condiments.

Condiment Ideas:

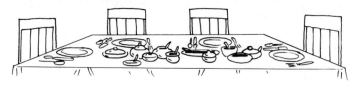

Raisins
Roasted Peanuts
Slivered almonds
Green pepper
Green onions
Chopped tomatoes

Sliced bananas
Yogurt
Sliced water chestnuts
Sliced cucumbers
Sliced radishes
Sliced red onion

Chris's Brown Rice Pilaf
Serves 4.

Chris is known for her grain dishes. When I ask her for dinner, I always have her bring "The starch."

1 cup raw brown rice
1/2 cup barley *or* wild rice
1 to 2 cups thinly sliced fresh mushrooms
4 cups homemade chicken broth
1/2 tsp. salt (optional)
1 tsp basil
1/2 cup fresh or frozen peas

Place all ingredients but the peas in a saucepan. Cook over moderate heat for 30 minutes. Add peas and cook for an additional 10 minutes.
Note: This is a complete protein: peas + brown rice.

Falsone White Sauce a la Yogurt
Serves 2.

A recipe like this one that calls for half butter and half oil (safflower, especially) is good in terms of cardiovascular health. The total amount of fat used, however, should be small, no more than 2 tsp. per serving.

1 Tblsp. oil
1 small clove garlic, minced
1/4 white onion, finely chopped
1 Tblsp. parsley
1 Tblsp. oil
1 Tblsp. butter
2 Tblsp. whole wheat flour
1/2 cup nonfat milk
1/4 cup white wine
1 cup low-fat or nonfat yogurt
Dash of black pepper

Saute garlic, onion, and parsley in oil. Turn heat to low and add butter, cooking until it melts. Add flour and stir until blended. Add milk and wine and stir until thick and smooth. Stirring constantly, blend in yogurt. Add pepper. Serve while hot. It's sensational over fish, chicken, steamed vegetables, or whole wheat pasta.

Variation: I add 1 cup of shredded, cooked chicken to the sauce and serve over whole wheat pasta. You can also use leftover turkey or shellfish.

Zucchini Lasagna

Serves 6.

This is a wonderful Italian dish. It's so low in fat and calories that you can come back for more and more and more! Your company will love it, too.

1 Tblsp. oil
2 large onions, finely chopped
4 garlic cloves, finely chopped
1 to 2 cups sliced fresh mushrooms
One 12-oz. can tomato sauce
One 12-oz. can tomato paste
One 16-oz. can tomatoes
1/2 cup white wine
1/2 tsp. pepper
1 tsp *each* oregano, basil, and Italian seasoning
4 to 5 zucchinis, sliced thinly *lengthwise* (these are the "noodles")
1 pint of low-fat cottage cheese
Parmesan cheese

Saute onion and garlic in oil in a nonstick skillet. Add mushrooms, tomato sauce, tomato paste, canned tomatoes, wine, and seasonings. Cut large tomato pieces into smaller ones. *Simmer for 1/2 to 1 hour.* In a 9x9-inch pan, arrange a layer of tomato mixture, then a layer of zucchini strips, then a layer of cottage cheese, then a sprinkling of parmesan cheese. Repeat layering process. Cover and bake in oven at 350°F for 3/4 to 1 hour. Bake uncovered for the last 10 minutes.

Eggplant-Mushroom Pasta Sauce
Serves 4.

This is a simple-to-prepare, yummy pasta topping. It will be one of your favorite vegetarian dishes.

1 Tblsp. olive oil
1 onion, chopped
1 eggplant, chopped (peeled or unpeeled)
4 Tblsp. chopped parsley
3 cloves garlic, minced
1/2 lb. fresh mushrooms, sliced
1/2 tsp. *each* thyme, rosemary, and oregano
4 fresh, ripe tomatoes, chopped
One 6-oz. can tomato paste
1 cup water
1 cup white wine
2 bay leaves
1/2 tsp. fennel seeds (essential)
1/8 tsp. cayenne pepper
Pepper to taste
Salt (optional)
2 Tblsp. red wine vinegar

Saute onion in oil. Add the rest of the ingredients, except for the vinegar. Simmer, covered, for 30 minutes. Remove lid and add vinegar. Cook, uncovered, for 50 minutes. Serve over whole wheat pasta.

Dee's Spaghetti Sauce
Serves 4-6.

Dee is losing LOTS of weight by staying on a low-fat food plan. She is also getting fit by exercising aerobically three to four times a week. Dee loves to cook, and is adapting all her recipes to include less fat, salt, and sugar. She *never* skimps on flavor.

2 onions, chopped
1 Tblsp. olive oil
1 lb. fresh mushrooms
Three 15-oz. cans tomato sauce
One 6-oz. can tomato paste
One 28-oz. can tomatoes
4 to 6 cloves garlic, minced
1 to 2 tsp. *each* basil and oregano
1/2 to 1 cup red wine
1 Tblsp. honey

Saute onions in olive oil in a nonstick pan. Add mushrooms and cook until soft. Puree tomatoes in blender. Add tomatoes and the rest of the ingredients and cook, covered, on a low heat for 1 to 3 hours. This sauce improves with age. Prepare a day in advance, if possible. Serve over whole wheat pasta and enjoy.

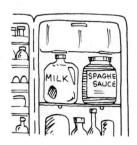

Joe's Spaghetti Sauce
Serves 4.

Joe is a physician who is a very warm, kind person. He enjoys a good meal after his workouts. This is one of his favorite dishes.

2 Tblsp. oil
2 carrots, chopped
1 onion, chopped
2 celery stalks, chopped
2 cloves garlic, diced
1 tsp. oregano
1 cup chicken broth
1 cup red wine
One 2-lb. can Italian tomatoes
2 Tblsp. parsley
1 tsp. basil
Salt and pepper to taste

Saute vegetables in oil. Add the rest of the ingredients and cook 40 minutes. Puree in blender or food processor. Serve over whole wheat, or whole wheat-soy noodles.

Tofu Sandwich Spread
Enough for 4 sandwiches.

For a refreshing change from the standard sandwich fillings, try this one and ENJOY!

1 cup tofu (1 cup = 1/2 lb.)
1 green onion, finely chopped
1 Tblsp. Ortega chilies, finely chopped
1/4 cup sunflower seeds
1 stalk celery, finely chopped
1 tsp. tamari soy sauce
1/4 tsp. cumin
1/4 tsp. paprika
1 clove garlic, minced
2 Tblsp. low-fat or nonfat plain yogurt

Mash tofu. Add onion, chilies, sunflower seeds, celery, seasonings, and spices. Stir in yogurt and mix until well blended. Serve on whole wheat bread with lettuce, sprouts, tomatoes, or any other favorite garnish.

Calvin's Yogurt

Even people who don't like yogurt LOVE this yogurt! Yogurt is an excellent source of calcium and protein. It makes a perfect light lunch, that has "staying power." (Calvin is a chemist who was awarded the Nobel Prize!)

3⅞ cups low-fat milk
1/2 cup nonfat noninstant milk powder
5 grams yogurt culture (yogourmet is packaged in 5-gram packs)

Blend milk and milk powder. Put in large pot with thermometer and heat to 150°F. When milk has reached this temperature, turn off immediately. It is very important to heat the milk to 150° (scalding temperature). This kills all offending growing bugs in the milk so that the yogurt culture has freedom to grow well. The heat also changes the molecular structure of the milk which aids in the culturing process.

Let cool to 110°F. Add culture packet with small whisk to distribute evenly. Pour into 1-quart canning jar with lid.

For an incubator use a crock lined with 2 inches of foam on bottom, sides and top. Put the crock in a draft-free location like a cold oven. This type of arrangement needs overnight incubation.

Variations: Add 1 to 2 teaspoons vanilla and 2 tablespoons honey to milk while cooking. This makes a slightly sweet yogurt for people who find plain yogurt too sour. You can substitute almond extract for the vanilla.

Salads

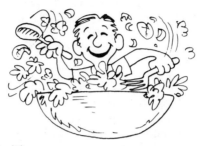

Basque Salad a la Tomas
Serves 4.

Tomas is a solar engineer who enjoys running in Strawberry Canyon in Berkeley. In his free time he does beautiful woodworking and cooks special dishes for his family. Here is one of his dinner salads.

1 cup fresh snow peas
1 head red leaf lettuce, cut in bit-sized pieces
2 cups fresh watercress
1 avocado, sliced
2 oranges, sliced
1 Tblsp. sesame seeds

Dressing:
2 Tbsp. oil
3 Tbsp. Vinegar
2 Tbsp. water
1 tsp. dry mustard
1 tsp. honey

Mix ingredients and shake WELL.
Note: For low-fat dressings, you always want the amount of oil to be equal to or less than the amount of liquid: vinegar, lemon juice, wine, or water.

Calamari Toss
Serves 6.

This dish can be served as a main meal for lunch or dinner. It's also an excellent addition to a Sunday Brunch.

2 Tblsp. olive oil
2 Tblsp. water
2 Tblsp. wine vinegar
1 to 2 Tblsp. lemon juice
Salt and pepper to taste
1/2 cucumber, thinly sliced
1/2 lb. mushrooms, thinly sliced
2 fresh tomatoes, thinly sliced
1½ lb. squid, cleaned and cut into rings
2 Tblsp. fresh parsley, finely chopped
Romaine lettuce

Combine oil, water, vinegar, lemon juice, and salt and pepper in a large bowl. Add vegetables and marinate for at least 1-1½ hours. Immerse squid rings in boiling water for 30 seconds. Overcooked squid is tough and chewy! It is important to cook it until just done—30 seconds is enough time. Drain squid and cook, then add marinade. Arrange on a bed of lettuce and sprinkle with parsley.

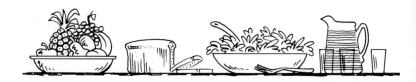

Mushroom Salad Dressing
Makes 1 quart.

Use a spicy tomato juice, such as Snappy Tom, for a hotter dressing. Serve over a tossed green salad.

1 lb. fresh mushrooms, sliced
1¼ cup tomato juice
1/3 cup white wine
1/4 tsp. crumbled oregano
2 Tblsp. finely chopped green onion
1 to 2 small garlic cloves, finely minced
1/8 tsp. black pepper

Rinse mushrooms and slice to make about 5-5½ cups. Place tomato juice, wine, oregano, onion, garlic, and pepper in a medium saucepan. Add mushrooms and bring to a boil. Reduce heat and simmer, covered, for 5 to 10 minutes. Pour into a bowl, cover, and refrigerate for at least 2 hours.

Soups

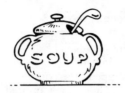

Casey's Black Bean Soup
Serves 4-6.

This soup is very high in iron. Black beans contain more iron than any other bean.

    2 cups black beans
    3 cups water
    5 cups water
    2 onions, cut in bite-sized pieces
    3 bay leaves
    1/2 tsp. thyme
    1/2 tsp. marjoram
    Garlic salt and pepper to taste

Soak beans in 3 cups water overnight. Drain off water. Put beans, 5 cups fresh water, and other ingredients in a pot. Bring to a boil then simmer for 1½ to 2 hours. Remove 1 cup of beans and blend in blender until smooth. Return to pot and mix in with the rest of the soup. Reheat and serve piping hot. Serve with a tossed green salad and whole-grain rolls.

Variations: Put 1 tablespoon sherry in each bowl. Put a dollop of low-fat plain yogurt on top.

Karole's Mushroom-Leek Soup
Serves 4-6.

This soup is healthy, low in fat and calories. Best of all, it tastes GREAT!

6 cups homemade stock (chicken, beef, or vegetable)
4 cups sliced fresh mushrooms
1 large onion, chopped
3 leeks, *thinly* sliced
1/4 cup brown rice
Salt and pepper to taste

Bring stock to a boil, add mushrooms, onion, leeks, and rice. Cook for 3/4 hour. Let cool slightly, then blend 2 to 3 cups in blender, doing small amounts at a time. Return to pot, reheat, and serve! This soup is very nice with a glob of yogurt and a spoonful of salsa sauce in the middle.

Tom's Baked Garlic and Vegetable Soup
Serves 4-6.

Here is an excellent low-calorie, low-fat soup. Don't let the amount of garlic throw you off; the baking transforms the taste. However, people know when Tom has eaten his soup!

2 cups diced fresh tomatoes
2 cups cooked beans (any kind)
5 zucchinis, sliced
2 large onions, sliced
1/2 bell pepper, diced
1½ cups white wine
5 to 6 cloves of garlic (the more, the better!)
1 bay leaf
1/2 tsp. salt (or to taste)
1/2 tsp. paprika
1 tsp. basil

Mix all ingredients in a large, oven-proof kettle, and bring to near boil on the stove. Then, put into a preheated 375°F oven for 1 to 1½ hours. Serve with a fresh-fruit salad and crunchy warm rolls.

Variation: A little broccoli or cauliflower cut into small pieces is also good in this soup.

Ayn's Scallop Soup
Serves 4 for a main dish; serves 6 as a first course.

Ayn is a gourmet cook. Everyone wants to come to her house for dinner. Not only does she prepare fabulous meals, but also she serves them in an elegant manner. You truly feel pampered while dining with Ayn.

2 Tblsp. oil
1½ cups finely chopped onion and leeks
4 medium tomatoes, chopped
4 cups liquid (fish stock, clam juice and water, or any mixture, with 1 cup of wine being one of the four cups).
1 large pinch saffron
1/2 cup tomato juice
One 8-oz. can tomato sauce
Tied in cheesecloth:
    pinch of thyme, 6 parsley sprigs, 1/2 tsp. basil
Salt and fresh ground pepper to taste
1 lb. fresh scallops

Cook leeks and onions slowly in oil for 5 to 6 minutes. Drain well. Put in a pot with the tomatoes, raise heat, and cook 3 to 4 minutes. Add all ingredients except the scallops. Bring to a boil, turn heat down, and simmer partially covered for 30 minutes. Add salt and pepper to taste.

Soak scallops in cold water for a few minutes. Cut into small slices. Bring soup base to a rapid boil, add scallops, and boil for 3 minutes. Check seasoning. Eat at once while hot!

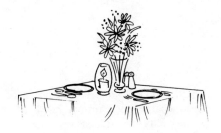

Legumes

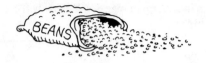

Spicy Bean Bowl
Serves 6.

This bean dish is spicy and flavorful. It can be served as a main dish or can be used as a burrito or tostada filling. The list of ingredients looks long, but you probably have most of them on hand.

1 Tblsp. oil
1½ large onions, chopped
5 cloves garlic, finely chopped
2 Tblsp. parsley, finely chopped
1¼ cup dried pinto beans, cooked
1/2 cup dried black beans, cooked
One 16-oz. can tomatoes
One 6-oz. can tomato paste
1 Tblsp. honey
2 bay leaves
1/4 tsp. paprika
1¼ tsp. cumin
1¼ tsp. basil
Pinch of salt
1/4 tsp. pepper
Pinch of cayenne

Saute onions, garlic, and parsley in oil in a nonstick skillet. Put all ingredients into a large pot. Simmer for 1/2 hour, adding water to thicken the mixture if necessary.

Hofbones' Curry
Serves 4.

Hofbones is a nickname for a dear friend who loves good food. This is one of his favorite dishes. (Hofbones is a jogger and is becoming a computer nut. He's also LEAN and MEAN!)

1 Tblsp. oil
1 large onion, chopped
2 cloves garlic, minced
1 cup fresh sliced mushrooms
1/2 cup uncooked brown rice
1½ tsp. curry powder
4 cups water
1/2 tsp. salt (optional)
2 Tblsp. lemon juice
1 cup uncooked lentils
1 bunch raw spinach, finely chopped
Low-fat or nonfat plain yogurt
Tomatoes sliced in wedges

Saute in the oil the onions, garlic, mushrooms, and rice. Add curry powder, water, salt, lemon juice, and lentils. Stir and simmer until tender, about 3/4 hour. Stir in spinach and serve immediately. Place a spoonful of yogurt in the center of the dish and garnish with fresh tomato slices.

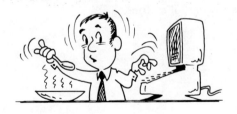

Tofu Chili
Serves 6 to 8.

This dish is good for a first try with tofu. It's tasty and failproof, and people always come back for more!

2 Tblsp. olive oil
2 medium onions, chopped
1 red bell pepper, chopped
1 green bell pepper, chopped
2 stalks celery, chopped
4 cloves garlic, minced
1 lb. firm tofu, cubed
1 tsp. basil
1 tsp. oregano
2 to 4 Tblsp. chili powder
1 tsp. cumin
6 large fresh tomatoes, chopped
One 15-oz. can tomato sauce
4 cups cooked pinto beans *or* a combination of kidney, pinto, and black or red beans
1/2 to 1 tsp. salt (optional)

Heat the oil over medium heat in a large saucepan. Add onions, peppers, celery, garlic, and tofu and saute until onions are transparent. Add herbs and spices and stir well. Mix in the tomatoes, tomato sauce, and cooked beans. Reduce heat, cover, and simmer for 1 hour. Serve with a large tossed green salad and whole wheat-cornmeal muffins.

Weahunt's Lentil Sauce
Serves 2 to 4.

Ms. Weahunt serves this sauce over pasta or a baked potato as a main dish.

2 tsp. oil
1 small onion, chopped
4 cloves garlic, minced
3 medium tomatoes, chopped
1/2 cup raw lentils
1 tsp. basil
1/2 cup white wine
One 8-oz. can tomato sauce
1 cup sliced fresh mushrooms
1/2 tsp. oregano
2 Tblsp. chopped parsley
1/2 tsp. thyme
Dash of tabasco sauce
2 cups cooked whole wheat pasta *or* 3 to 4 baked potatoes

In a nonstick pan, cook onion and garlic briefly in oil. Add all other ingredients except pasta or potatoes. Bring to a boil, reduce heat, cover, and simmer for 3/4 hour. Cook the pasta or baked potatoes and top with sauce.

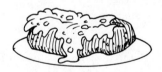

Vegetables

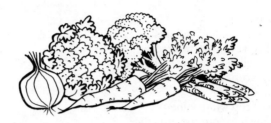

Cauliflower—Carrot Puree
Serves 4.

Vegetables purees are excellent when they are served together side by side for color and flavor contrast. You can puree almost any vegetable: spinach, asparagus, yellow squash, zucchini, and so on. Make little strips of purees on each person's plate—impressive!

    1 small cauliflower, chopped
    4 medium carrots, sliced
    1/4 cup low-fat plain yogurt
    Salt (optional), pepper, and nutmeg to taste

Steam vegetables for 10 to 15 minutes or until tender. Puree in blender, along with yogurt. Add salt and pepper to taste and a pinch of nutmeg.

Potato-Rutabaga Puree
Serves 4.

3 medium red potatoes, chopped
1 medium rutabaga, chopped
1/4 cup yogurt
Salt (optional), pepper, and nutmeg to taste

Steam vegetables for 15 to 20 minutes or until tender. Puree *lightly* in blender, along with yogurt. Add salt and pepper to taste, along with a little nutmeg.

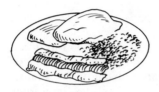

Italian Potato Pot
Serves 4-6.

This is a hassle-free dish that can accompany any seafood or chicken dish. It is very popular and will go fast!

Potatoes, diced
Onions, sliced
Fresh green beans
Fresh tomatoes, sliced
Fresh mushrooms, sliced
1/4 cup chicken stock

In a casserole dish place a layer of sliced potatoes, cover it with a layer of sliced onions, next with a layer of fresh green beans, followed by a layer of sliced tomatoes, topped with a layer of sliced mushrooms. Repeat layering until the casserole dish is filled to the top. Pour in the chicken stock and bake at 350° F for 3/4 to 1 hour. Enjoy!

Pear and Zucchini Stir
Serves 4.

This sounds like a weird combination, but it's excellent!

2 cups fresh pears, chopped (2 pears)
3 cups zucchini, sliced
2 tsp. olive oil
1/2 cup onion, sliced
1 clove garlic, minced
1/4 tsp. salt
1/4 tsp. oregano
1/4 tsp. basil
1/4 tsp. lemon peel

Cut fruit. Slice zucchini into 1/3-inch-thick, coin-like pieces. Heat oil in skillet and add onion, garlic, salt, and herbs. Add zucchini and lemon peel and fry for 5 minutes. Add pears and steam covered another 5 minutes. Serve immediately, while hot.

Spinach with Pear
Serves 4.

This is a wonderful dish, simple but elegant.

1 tsp. butter
2 green onions, chopped
1 lb. fresh spinach, well cleaned
1 ripe pear, finely chopped
1/4 tsp. nutmeg (freshly grated, if possible)
Salt and pepper to taste

Melt butter in skillet. Add green onions and saute for a few minutes. Add other ingredients. Cook, stirring constantly, until just heated through.

Mustard

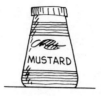

Linda's Mustard Sauce
Serves 8 to 10.

Linda is an excellent cook. She has also lost 30 pounds by eating a low-fat diet and jogging regularly!

1 medium-sized onion
1 bunch green onions
1 stalk celery
2 cloves garlic
1/4 cup parsley
1 Tblsp. paprika
1/4 tsp. cayenne
1/4 cup oil
1/2 cup Dijon mustard
2 Tblsp. lemon juice
2 Tblsp. vinegar
1 Tblsp. Worcestershire sauce
1/4 tsp. Tabasco sauce

Combine all ingredients and puree in food processor or blender. Allow sauce to sit for 24 hours. Serve with seafood or chicken.

Patti's Christmas Mustard
Makes 2 cups.

At Christmas time Patti makes this mustard for all her special friends. It is truly the best gift she could give, because it is wonderful. Try it and you'll agree!

1½ cups dry white wine (Chenin Blanc)
1 large onion, chopped
3 cloves garlic, minced
One 4-oz. can dry mustard
2 Tblsp. honey
1 Tblsp. oil
1 tsp. salt (optional)
Few drops Tabasco sauce

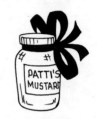

Combine wine, onion, and garlic in a small saucepan, heat to boiling, then lower heat and simmer for 5 minutes. Strain and let cool. Slowly pour wine mixture into dry mustard in a saucepan, beating constantly with a wire whip until very smooth. Blend honey, oil, salt, and Tabasco sauce into mustard mixture. Heat slowly, stirring constantly until mixture thickens. Cool. Pour into container (not metal). Chill 2 days to blend. Keep refrigerated.

Appetizers

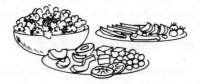

Ceviche

Makes 8 to 10 appetizers or 6 main servings.

I'm always searching for appeitzers that are low in fat and sugar and that taste yummy. This is just the dish. It calls for raw fish as its main ingredient: halibut, snapper, cod, fresh tuna, scallops, or shrimp. The cubed fish is "cooked" in lime juice and then combined with a spicy sauce. Serve ceviche as an appetizer with whole wheat pita bread as an exotic way to begin an enjoyable meal.

2 cups cubed fish (preferably two types)
1 cup lime juice
1 cup chopped peeled tomatoes
1/4 cup chopped green onion
3 Tblsp. olive oil
1 Tblsp. dry white wine
1 Tblsp. white vinegar
1 Tblsp. chili salsa (your favorite hot sauce)
1½ Tblsp. minced parsley
1/4 tsp. oregano
Dash salt and pepper
1 cup tomato juice (optional)

Place cubed fish in glass dish. The fish must be cut into *very* small pieces so that the lime juice can "cook" it thoroughly. If juice does not cover fish, add more. Cover and let stand for 3 hours at room temperature. Drain fish and rinse in water, then dry well. Mix other ingredients together. Add fish to sauce. Chill.

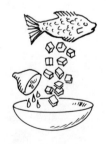

Toasted Tortilla Triangles
Makes 72.

12 corn tortillas
Morton's Lite Salt (optional)

Cut tortilla into 6 pie wedge-shaped pieces. Spread out half of the tortilla wedges on a baking sheet and salt lightly. Place the baking sheet in the pre-heated 400°F oven for 10 minutes. Turn each triangle over and return to oven for 3 to 4 more minutes. Remove the wedges and place the second half of the tortillas on the baking sheet and repeat the process.

Note: 6 tortilla chips = 70 calories.

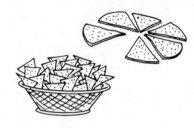

Chris's Apple Supreme
Serves 4

Chris often serves this to company. No one has a clue that it is low in fat.

3 cups apples
1/3 cup raisins
1/4 cup honey
2 Tblsp. whole wheat flour
2 cups apple juice
1/4 cup nonfat milk
1/2 tsp. cinnamon
1/4 tsp. nutmeg
1/4 tsp. ground cloves
Slivered almonds
Ricotta cheese

Wash and cut apples into bite-sized pieces. Place apples, juice, spices, and honey into a pot and cook for 5 minutes. Add milk to flour and stir to a smooth paste. Add to apples. Cook until just thickened, about 2 minutes. Remove from heat and spoon warm mixture into serving dishes. Top with a dab of ricotta cheese and slivered almonds. Enjoy!

Chris's Apple Supreme
Serves 4.

Chris often serves this to company. No one has a clue that it is low in fat!

3 cups apples
1/3 cup raisins
1/4 cup honey
2 Tblsp. whole wheat flour
2 cups apple juice
1/4 cup nonfat milk
1/2 tsp. cinnamon
1/4 tsp. nutmeg
1/4 tsp. ground cloves
Slivered almonds
Ricotta cheese

Wash and cut apples into bite-sized pieces. Place apples, juice, spices, and honey into a pot and cook for 5 minutes. Add milk to flour and stir to a smooth paste. Add to apples. Cook until just thickened, about 2 minutes. Remove from heat and spoon warm mixture into serving dishes. Top with a dab of ricotta cheese and slivered almonds. Enjoy!

BIBLIOGRAPHY

Black, Helen. *The Berkeley Co-op Food Book: Eat Better and Spend Less.* Palo Alto, Calif.: Bull Publishing Co., 1980.

Mellin, Laurel. *Weight Management Program for Adolescents.* San Francisco: Balboa Publishing, 1980.

Farquhar, John W. *The American Way of Life Need Not Be Hazardous to Your Health.* New York: W.W. Norton, 1978.

Brody, Jane E. *Jane Brody's Nutrition Book: A Lifetime Guide to Good Eating for Better Health and Weight Control.* New York: W.W. Norton, 1981.

Fox, Edward L., and Mathews, Donald K. *The Physiological Basis of Physical Education and Athletics.* Philadelphia: Saunders College Publishing, 1981.

Zohman, Lenore R., M.D. *Run for Life.* Connecticut Mutual Life Insurance Co., 1978.

Eating For A Healthy Heart. American Heart Association, Alameda County Chapter, Oakland, Calif., 1981.

Wood, Peter. *The California Diet.* Mountain View, Calif.: Anderson World Books, Inc., 1983.